SEND IN THE CLONES

~ Marvin Ginsburg, MD ~

DEDICATION

To my daughter Carol who I miss
every day but lives in my heart

ACKNOWLEDGEMENT

I am extremely grateful to my son Mark for his advice,
encouragement and technical assistance.
I want to express my heartfelt gratitude to all of the
dedicated nurses that I worked with at Palmdale Regional
Medical Center during my many years of hospital practice,
without whom I could not have become the doctor that I
aspired to be.

— 1 —

THE INTERNSHIP

D octor Sharon Dell walked into the room and gazed at the tiny figure of Charlie Baker lying so peacefully upon the small bed. The gentle sobbing of his parents, who were sitting by the window, broke the oppressive silence. Sharon knew that it would only be a matter of hours before Charlie would leave this world for a better one. She was convinced all children go to heaven when they die, but it didn't make her feel any better about it. Mrs. Baker interrupted her thoughts.

"Why is this happening?" she asked.

Sharon remained silent for a moment as she desperately struggled for an answer. "I don't have an answer," she murmured, swallowing hard to overcome her tears while placing her arms around Mona Baker.

"I'm so sorry," she said in a whisper, and walked slowly out of the room, wiping tears from her eyes.

Later that evening, Sharon returned to Charlie's room carrying a small package. She unwrapped a small music box and placed it at the bedside. Charlie loved music and had commented on the music box Sharon kept on her desk. During one clinic visit, while Charlie and his mother were waiting in her office for the lab results, Sharon was pleased to find that Charlie had become enchanted with the device. When she returned an hour later, Mona Baker told her that Charlie has been able to take a nap for the first time without a battle. There was no doubt the music had cast a soothing balm over Charlie with its gentle melodies. Even though she wasn't certain Charlie could still hear, she was moved to bring the box for him.

It was already 8 p.m., and she couldn't bring herself to leave and go home to her lonely apartment. She asked herself, *Why can't I be spared the pain of a child's death? How will I cope, or better yet, can I ever cope with it?* She walked out of the room and headed for the doctors' dressing room. Pouring herself a cup of coffee, she thought, *Why do we have these god-awful Styrofoam cups? They're so small and they only hold five good sips.* Sharon knew her thoughts were ridiculous, but she also knew they were purposeful. It was easier to overcome depression when she focused on unimportant minutia. Ever since surgical residency, she'd realized her inability to remain objective about her patients. It was always a major effort for her to remain detached, to separate emotional feelings from the hard clinical disease. Whenever a patient became gravely ill or died, she felt the onslaught of depression. The guilt she perceived was always there to be reckoned with as well. She felt accountable whenever a patient died. Over the years, she'd learned how to desensitize herself to these emotions, but lately it had become more difficult than ever. Sharon considered the reason for this and concluded it was because of the increased number of surgeries she was now performing. Even though she took immense delight in sharing in the successful transplant outcomes, it wasn't enough. As a matter of fact, it was inconsequential—it all seemed so meaningless. A new life, only to be cut short by a birth defect, disease, or accident, was just not right.

She felt responsible for all patients whom she cared for because of the psychodynamics of her own past. Sharon had finally understood that her own emotional conflicts had their seeds sown in her early childhood. Her mother had been a nurse and had immersed Sharon with her deep compassion at an early age by telling her stories about her work. When an unhappy hospital event caused her mother emotional distress, she related the detailed events to Sharon. Never did she realize that seeds of guilt and despair were being planted in her daughter's innocent mind. Sharon soaked up the fascinating tales of sickness, death, and sorrow, and suppressed them into her subconscious. There were too many things her young mind was unable to grasp, and this was the way she dealt with things that frightened her. The suppression of these childhood stories never surfaced until she was forced to deal with similar events and circumstances in her own professional life, and then it all began again.

The first time it happened, she was on the pediatric rotation of her internship. Sharon loved kids and was eagerly looking forward to the three-month rotation. She was assigned the care of twelve children on the pediatric ward at the University Hospital's Bayside campus. She found her work with children both exciting and rewarding, not to mention the enormous challenge each case presented. Finding the cause of children's illnesses and rendering the cure was only the first step. Her gratification came when she looked upon the child's face. It always amazed her how children wore their illnesses on their faces. It certainly wasn't that way with adults. Kids hadn't accomplished the feat of deception and therefore were unable to hide their illness, whereas adults were well trained in concealing their feelings and emotions. Sharon was strongly considering the specialty of pediatrics for her lifelong profession until the day she was called to the Emergency Room to admit a four-year-old boy with acute leukemia. The family pediatrician, Dr. Homer Trent, had suspected the diagnosis. He had been examining Paul Kimbert a week before in his office for a routine checkup when he discovered a severe anemia. The blood had also revealed many immature forms of white blood cells characteristic of leukemia. He was admitted to have further testing and a diagnostic bone marrow examination. If the diagnosis were confirmed, chemotherapy would then follow.

Sharon took a detailed history from Mr. and Mrs. Kimbert and examined Paul. She learned of Paul's nosebleeds and painful right ear. There was a history of black and blue marks, which had spontaneously occurred over the last few weeks. He showed evidence of recent weight loss, appeared very pale and weak, and didn't show much interest in his surroundings. Her examination disclosed a middle ear infection, and there were enlarged lymph nodes in the neck and groin. There was bruising noted all over his body and his liver was enlarged.

She wrote the initial admitting orders and spoke with the parents. They were devastated by the suspected disease but were still not easily accepting of the diagnosis. Sharon couldn't suppress her feelings of compassion and spent much time explaining the need for the bone marrow examination as well as the disease itself. She even talked at length about the great successes with new chemotherapy techniques.

The following day, the pathologist confirmed the diagnosis of acute leukemia, and Sharon informed the family. At first their reaction was one of denial, which overshadowed rationality, but after extensive explanation, Mr. and Mrs. Kimbert eventually acquiesced and agreed to chemotherapy. Sharon was long suffering in her explanation of chemotherapy as she explained the way the drugs interfered with the growth of the leukemic cells along with the inherent risks associated with them. She told the parents that the drugs might not have any effect on the disease, or could cause serious side effects or severe infections. She explained that the infections that usually occurred did so because of suppressed immunity brought about by the disease as well as the drugs. Sharon explained that in most cases, these opportunistic infections were cured by the armamentarium of antibiotics that were now available. Furthermore, she informed them that on occasion, these newer antibiotics failed and the patient succumbed to the infection. Sharon met with the parents over two days and answered all their questions. As expected, she repeated most of her dialogue many times until they at last agreed to the chemotherapy. She had been through an intense brainwashing and thought, *This is what a debriefing must be like. Just like a computer, I've downloaded all my acquired knowledge of acute leukemia to the Kimberts.* Sharon agreed to meet with them once more to answer any final questions they might have.

During the two days of discussions, it became necessary to give Paul several blood transfusions to build him up for the chemotherapy. Mr. and Mrs. Kimbert had finally given their written consent, and the administration of the poisons began. Throughout the drug regimen, Paul remained in guarded condition and eventually failed the induction course of chemotherapy. His platelets, responsible for clotting, along with the red blood cells, remained pitifully low, and despite all the aggressive attempts initiated to stymie the growth of the leukemic cells, the drugs failed. Paul died quietly during his sleep on a night Sharon was working. She was called to the bedside by the nurse to perform the perfunctory task of certifying Paul's passport that he had indeed left this earth. At his bedside, she sat and sobbed. Paul's face was peaceful at last, and it was right at that moment she developed the guilt.

Sharon had convinced the parents to give consent for the chemotherapy, but perhaps if she hadn't, Paul would still have been alive. If she hadn't, maybe the leukemia would have entered spontaneous remission, for it had been known to happen before. If she hadn't done such a good job in convincing the parents that chemotherapy was the proper thing to do, the drugs wouldn't have killed Paul's red blood cell and platelet production. Sharon sobbed hysterically and refused to wipe the tears away. She deserved to suffer and feel the guilt; it was all her fault.

She couldn't sleep that night or the next, becoming more

despondent until she was unable to function. Her friends noticed her demeanor and took her to the psychiatric clinic. After three months of psychiatric counseling five times a week, Sharon finally understood the mechanics of her emotions and learned how to cope with them. The trick was to distance herself from the families and to deal only with the patient in an objective manner.

Sharon awakened to find she had fallen asleep at the desk in the doctor's dressing room. The coffee had grown cold, so she poured herself a new cup. Suddenly she felt the need for compassion and understanding. She knew where she could get it, and left the hospital. This was her weekend off the call schedule, so it would be easy for her to visit her father in Auburn, California.

~2~

TALKING IT OVER

D r. Karl Dell was a specialist in the field of Internal Medicine who had been practicing actively until three years ago, when he declared to himself that he was semi-retired. After working fifteen hours a week in a medical clinic, he became bored, and to no one's surprise went to work for the state of California as a medical inspector for the Department of Corporations. The DOC was charged with the oversight of all aspects of managed care. This included the health maintenance organizations (HMOs), the medical groups delivering care for the HMOs, and the hospitals that provided any medical care for patients on an HMO medical insurance plan.

Karl loved his new position, although it didn't pay exorbitantly. The job required that he inspect various medical facilities, medical groups, hospitals, and clinics, and even the main offices of the HMOs. This afforded him the opportunity to travel throughout the state and render his opinion as to the quality of care at the facilities he inspected.

The best part of the job was that he could set his own

hours. Because of the pay scale, the state only had one other physician to assist with the work. Karl was convinced the Peter Principle was alive and well, and to that end he refused to give up hands-on medical practice for fear of losing his clinical abilities. In order for him to evaluate others for quality of care as well as issues such as the appropriateness of procedures and proper utilization, he had to be doing these things himself. This gave him the proper perspective and made him an excellent inspector.

Needless to say, Karl loved his job and had found his niche. The other love in his life was Sharon, his only child. Karl's wife had died ten years before from a protracted illness, which had left him devastated and extremely lonely. His life was consumed by Sharon and his devotion to the care of the sick. He had deep compassion for his patients, compassion that was easily seen. At age sixty-two, he was still physically fit, with the exception of the ten pounds of extra weight he carried. His beard was trim, and its salt-and-pepper coloring matched his curly hair. Every day he jogged three miles or more, and he did a light workout in his own home on a Universal weight system. Sharon had a very special relationship with her father, which had developed since childhood. He had become the only one she ever trusted with her innermost thoughts, and he, in return, treasured the relationship.

When she walked through the door, he knew immediately her soul was heavily burdened.

"Hi Dad, how are you?" she said, trying desperately to muster a smile.

"All is well with me, my beautiful daughter, but not with you. Your face is a giveaway."

"You read my mind as usual, Dad. I'm in the pits."

"Why don't we sit down like old times and talk?" he said, as he hugged her close to him.

Sharon loved it when he did that. She felt so secure and protected from the world, just like when she was a child. The only difference now was that Dad couldn't make her sorrow leave like he used to then. "Sure Dad, I'd like that very much. It's so hard keeping things bottled up when you're hurting so much."

Karl gazed at his daughter's large, sad, hazel eyes. She so reminded him of his wife, but was slightly taller at five-seven. Her light brown hair draped her shoulders and she was a trim 117 pounds. She was one of those lucky women who always looked great and never had to work at it.

"Why don't we sit at the kitchen table the way we used to? I'll put on a pot of coffee just like old times."

"I don't have anyone I can trust with my feelings," said Sharon.

"Well you do now, so have at it dear."

"I just lost another patient," said Sharon, wiping a tear from her eye. Karl looked at her face and immediately wanted to assume her sorrow. It reminded him of the time when she'd become depressed as an intern—in the end, she had overcome her despondency and was able to complete the internship.

She had been indecisive about her future, though, and after six months had settled on surgery as her profession.

Sharon reasoned that surgery would allow her to limit her emotional involvement with patients. Her job would be to cut and cure and return the patient to the referring doctor for handholding. It seemed all other medical specialties honed in on the doctor-patient relationship, which by inference meant personal involvement to some degree. She would convert and direct all her emotional energies to the technical aspects of surgery.

Throughout her surgical residency, she sharpened her skills, and each year it became easier to divorce her feelings from the patient. Her life was shrouded in procedural applications and diagnostics. The other specialists, who left her to concentrate entirely on her art, referred all her patients. These patients had their own doctors who were their confidants. She was able to remain aloof from them and derive full satisfaction from her surgeries. The reward of seeing the patients leave the hospital, usually in much better condition than on arrival, was all she required.

Over the four years of surgical training, Sharon managed to build a wall about the patients and to confine her involvement to the pathology alone, but the first two years of the residency demanded that she spend more time with them than the last two years. During the first year, she was responsible for the basic workup of the surgical candidate and following the chief resident on his daily hospital rounds. She rapidly acquired the skills of physical diagnosis and how to use the more elaborate diagnostic modalities. Although she was well liked by her professors and supervising residents, they all recognized how she never became close to any patient.

In the third and fourth year of the residency program, she spent more time in the operating room and less on the floors with patients, which made her life easier. The chairman of the Department of Surgery, who had made the selection upon the receipt of glowing reports of Sharon's surgical abilities, appointed her as the Chief Resident in Surgery for her final year.

She had now been duly noted as a rising star. All the "good" surgical cases were reserved for her knife, and she also demonstrated her abilities as a teacher, since she was now responsible for the teaching of all the junior residents. Sometime during the first three months of that year, she had a rude awakening as she realized she didn't know what she would do at the end of her final year in training. Sharon thought about all the offers for practice she'd received, but they only served as a nidus of anxiety, which grew bigger each day. There was something missing—a void in her heart. The emotional gratification she derived from her surgery still wasn't enough. Sharon missed the children. For four long years she had desperately tried to escape her desire to comfort children. Suddenly it occurred to her that she might have her cake and eat it too. She could fulfill this insatiable desire to help children and not become emotionally involved, if she limited her surgery to the pediatric age group. Yes, she would train further to become a pediatric surgeon.

Sharon applied for and was accepted to a two-year pediatric surgical fellowship training program at the University Teaching Hospital. She tackled her new learning experience with renewed vigor and was brilliant.

The two years passed swiftly, and again she found herself unable to decide her future direction. She loved performing pediatric surgery and the gratification of the job well done, but she still felt emptiness. Something was lacking—she wanted to contribute her talents toward something special. She thought she should be able to contribute to children something that they could not acquire from all the other surgeons. It just so happened that the Hospital of San Bernardino was initiating an organ transplant surgical fellowship training program. The program was under the leadership of one of the most renowned surgeons in the world, Dr. Jacob Bailey, a full professor and chairman of the newly developed department that was under the auspices of Southern California University. She knew she had found it at last—the missing piece of the puzzle. There were two openings in the program and twenty applicants, but Sharon was easily accepted to the two-year program.

She became an expert in both adult and pediatric organ transplantations. During her training, she learned the details of kidney and liver transplant surgery, as well as of intestinal and pancreatic transplantation, and when she completed the program, she had no difficulty in choosing her direction. Sharon applied for a full-time faculty position as Assistant Chief of the rapidly growing Transplant Surgery Department at Southern California University. At the age of thirty-five, she was the youngest assistant department chief in any program throughout the United States. For the next two-and-a-half years, she operated five days a week and eventually began to feel the pressure arising from the lack of donor organs. She was deeply concerned by the pediatric donor supply.

She had told her dad previously that the majority of her cases were adults and her pediatric patients were succumbing before coming to surgery for lack of replacement organs. Now, Karl was startled by her voice. "I'm sorry Sharon, I guess I was daydreaming a bit."

"Dad, I don't think I can take any more of this. For every pediatric patient I save in surgery, ten die because of the lack of donor organs. I guess I need a long vacation."

"Sharon, you are taking the responsibilities of the world on your shoulders. It isn't your fault you don't have the organs. Take solace in the fact that you cure ninety-five percent of the patients you are able to operate upon. Your talents and dedication have allowed hundreds of children to live normal lives. Be content with that."

"I can't, Dad. I feel the loss of children's lives even though I am not intimately involved with them in their pre-operative care. I see the child once to evaluate them for an organ transplant surgery, and that's all I need to mentally connect. It becomes impossible for me to forget that I never got the chance to give them a new liver or kidney. I always know that we weren't quick enough when the child fails to show for their three-month follow-up visit at my clinic."

Karl went to the stove and poured two cups of coffee, then brought them to the table. While pouring, he thought for a moment and decided to tell Sharon about The Wickford Medical Center Hospital.

"My dear, organs must be donated to the University Hospital, but in the private sector, there are no restrictions as to the source of the donors."

"I don't follow you."

"It is a well-kept secret known only by a select few that The Wickford Medical Center acquires organs from donors who sell them in South America, Mexico, and other third-world countries."

"I'm shocked, I can't believe it," said Sharon, shaking her head in bewilderment while gesturing with outstretched hands.

"It's true, so help me. According to the California State statistics on transplant surgery last year, TWMC performed thirty-eight hundred organ transplants."

"Unbelievable! We only did one thousand transplants at The University Children's Hospital Center."

"That proves my point. You can't get the organs because the university's rules prohibit the purchase of them. In the private hospital sector, there are no such regulations. Obviously TWMC has plenty of money, since they pay upwards of fifteen thousand dollars for each organ."

"How can they recapture the price of the organ? The surgery and hospital fees are so god-awful as is, even without a charge for the organ."

"I don't know that answer, but I do know that what I told you is true."

"How can you be so sure?"

"Let me tell you a story, Sharon," said Karl as he sipped his coffee. "About a year ago, I became somewhat bored and decided I needed to be busier, so I got a job with The Department of Corporations for the State of California. The DOC is the regulatory agency for all managed care companies in the state. I was hired to examine specific records of managed care patients at various hospitals. Six months ago, I was sent to TWMC to perform such a medical audit, where I spent one day reviewing the medical records computer data to determine the nature of high-volume operative procedures. I expected to be reviewing medical records of abdominal surgeries for the previous year, but instead I was shocked to find the high-volume cases were transplant surgeries. After reviewing sixty cases, I found that each potential surgical case was operated upon within four weeks of the time the decision to perform transplant surgery was made. I became very suspicious about two issues. How was it possible that a hundred percent of patients who needed donor organs got them, and how could all the organs be supplied in a timely fashion?"

"What did you do, Dad?" "I reported these findings to the DOC, and after a review, it was determined the hospital had broken no law and it was within their right to procure donor organs for a price if they chose to do so. I interviewed the chief of the transplant program, Dr. Gary Moss, who was very frank about their acquisitions. He has been the chairman of the transplant section for five years and told me they are looking for qualified transplant surgeons to add to their staff. At that time, he was the only transplant surgeon, and he was seeking to find another one desperately. When I told him you were my daughter, he loosened up somewhat and spoke about you with great respect. You are well known in the field and I, of course, was very flattered. He convinced me to ask you to call him, but I didn't tell you about it. I thought you were happy in your present position—had I known otherwise, I would have told you sooner."

"Maybe I should give him a call. What have I got to lose? If there is still a position available, I would welcome the change and the opportunity to save more kids." Sharon's mood improved immediately with the knowledge that a possibility for change loomed in the future. She decided she would make contact with Doctor Moss the next week.

After that, Karl and his daughter reminisced about the past and eventually got into a discussion about the state of medicine as related to managed care.

"Do you think TWMC will be affected much by managed care?" asked Sharon. "There should only be one level of medical care regardless of financial class," she added.

"True, but in the real world, it is controlled by physicians," said Karl.

"The problem is that the physician group that delivers the care becomes the gatekeeper and makes all the decisions concerning a patient's care."

"But that is what always occurred before the days of the HMO," said Karl.

"That may be so, but before the HMO days, doctors were not influenced by financial gain," retorted Sharon.

"Sharon, you are being very naive. If you believe doctors always made clinical decisions based only on the patient's need, you are sadly mistaken."

"I don't follow you."

"Look, doctors have had ownership in hospitals, labs, pharmacies, radiology, CAT scans, MRIs, Physical therapy centers, home health care companies, and every imaginable type of medically related business in the world. Do you believe all those doctors always referred their patients on the basis of clinical indication only?" asked Karl.

"Are you telling me that physicians were motivated by financial remuneration?"

"Yes. I am telling you that people are human, and when they see an opportunity to feather their own bed, they will. It becomes easier to rationalize the need or indication for a test or procedure when you know that you'll gain financially from it."

"Certainly these were only few and far between in their occurrence."

"Sharon, I suppose these 'opportunities' happened often enough to classify them as not rare happenings, but certainly not very common either. The feds clamped down on many of them over the years with respect to physicians providing any services other than the practice of medicine within the Medicare program. The law mandated a full disclosure of any financial involvement by the doctor or his family in any business that deals with a Medicare recipient. There have been many doctors convicted of fraud and other federal violations dealing with 'self referrals.'"

"I guess, then, there isn't a whole lot of difference between doctors' financial incentives then and now," said Sharon. "That's exactly my point with a slight modification. They used to be involved with over-utilization of procedures and medical resources, but today they are involved in underutilization. The failure to perform a procedure or to properly hospitalize a patient when clinically necessary is a tool by which they save money; therefore, more is left in the pot for them. The capitation dollar will only stretch so far. If costs can be reduced on the care of the patient, there is more left over in profit."

"What about the proficiency of the doctor who works for a group with a managed care contract?" asked Sharon. "Do you think they are of the same caliber?"

"Medical groups have been forced into hiring all types of doctors to do primary care or what we used to call general practice. Today we see obstetricians, surgeons, and specialists from all walks of medicine performing primary care. The market forces provoked it, because there were never enough primary care docs available. The upward surge in California HMO business required that medical groups have enough primary care docs to see the everyday, bread-and-butter medical patient. The problem now is that these doctors are not trained in the basics of general or family practice, and they miss many illnesses. Late diagnoses lead to untoward outcomes and dissatisfaction. In my opinion, this is the basis for the majority of complaints in managed care. The news media loves to place blame on the doctor and point to these failures as a direct result of doctors' greed. The failure to act appropriately and swiftly, influenced by the fact they can save a buck, is really a rare occurrence and is no different than it was before the advent of the HMO."

It was getting late, and Sharon was exhausted. She said goodnight to Karl and went to her bedroom to retire. The next morning, after a leisurely breakfast and catching up on the latest world news, she departed for home.

She thought about her talk with her father and marveled

again at the fact that she now felt so much better. She had hope and could see things clearer now. Her intuition told her she would be leaving San Bernardino Hospital. Somehow, the boring drive south on Interstate 5 passed quickly.

～3～

MAKING A CHANGE
FOR THE BETTER

S haron's schedule was light on Monday morning, so at 10
a.m. she found the time to call Doctor Gary Moss at
TWMC.

"Doctor Moss, good morning, this is Sharon Dell at
Children's in San Bernardino."

"Yes Sharon, how are you?"

"I'm fine, Doctor Moss. I am calling you to inquire if
you still have a position open in transplant surgery?" she said
while crossing her fingers on her right hand.

"Why yes, as a matter of fact we do. We are desperately
in need of someone to direct our new pediatric transplant
program. We are about to bring on two young pediatric surgeons for a two-year fellowship training program in pediatric
transplant surgery. Now we need a chief of the department.
Are you interested?"

Sharon could hardly believe her ears. This was even
more than she had hoped for. Transplantation surgery was

not yet a subspecialty of pediatric surgery. All transplant surgeons performed their art on both adults and children, with the emphasis on the former group. It was difficult to gain enough experience on the pediatric group, because most of their diseases that led to transplant surgery were congenital and not acquired illnesses like those seen in the adult group. This obviously led to a diminished number of such cases for training purposes. If a pediatric program was developed, it could become a referral center, and the number of pediatric cases would be large. This was what a program needed, so that younger surgeons could gain proper training.

"I am interested in the position," she said rapidly.

"That's great, Sharon. You don't mind if I call you Sharon, do you?"

"No, not at all. As a matter of fact, I prefer you do."

"Fine, please call me Gary. I would like you to FedEx your curriculum vitae to me as quickly as possible. Our hospital board meets next week and I want to present your qualifications to them. Can you meet me this week for an interview, and I will show you around the hospital?"

"What about Thursday at two o'clock," asked Sharon.

"That will be fine. I'll look for you then."

Sharon's spirit soared. She'd never considered the possibility of becoming the chief of the new Department of Pediatric Transplant Surgery. It was almost too good to be true. For the next two-and-a-half days, she seemed to walk on air.

Finally, the day arrived, and Sharon drove to TWMC for her interview.

"Doctor Moss, I am Sharon Dell."

"Very happy to meet you, Sharon. Your reputation pre-cedes you." Moss interviewed Sharon for close to an hour and then took her on a tour of the facility. She was amazed at the diagnostic armamentarium as well as the rest of the facility. She discovered that the center had the major Tertiary Hospital contract for the two largest HMO companies in the state, meaning all patients in any other hospital in Southern California requiring transfer to a higher level of care were referred to TWMC. In addition to the increase in patient cen-sus that resulted from this, the HMOs also paid a higher daily bed rate to the hospital. Sharon was told that this agreement was made to allow the HMOs to advertise that TWMC was the tertiary center. The sales force capitalized on this, and employers were convinced to purchase the HMO insurance for their employees. Southern California industry was now paying strict attention to the provisions of health plans, and when all was said and done, the costs were pretty much the same. By contracting with these plans, they had the added insurance that in the advent of a devastating illness, the pa-tient would be referred to the finest medical center. In addi-tion, TWMC had already acquired a reputation for its highly successful transplant program. Now that it could boast the beginning of the new pediatric transplant program, the large employers were sold on these HMOs. The bottom line, Moss told Sharon, was that the hospital received more patients and more money for their care, and the HMOs sold more medi-cal insurance, which covered any potential financial downside for them.

She was hired for the position of Chief of the Pediatric Transplant Department at TWMC. In this capacity, she was promoted to full professor at the University of San Diego Medical School. The university ran the teaching program for interns and residents at TWMC, which made Sharon responsible for developing and directing the teaching program.

She was thrilled with her new position and its tenet responsibilities. In her capacity, she was also required to perform transplant surgery on adults as well. She knew it would be a while before she became too busy with pediatric cases to operate on adults.

Sharon had been at her new position for only five weeks when she was given the go-ahead to initiate the new pediatric transplant surgery program. From nowhere seemed to come young patients to be evaluated for the liver and kidney transplantation program. The HMO referrals were directed to her from as far away as Sacramento. She evaluated fifteen patients in only two short weeks and placed them all on the waiting list for donor livers and kidneys, never in her wildest dreams suspecting that the first transplant would happen in four weeks.

After the first case, all the others followed rapidly. No patient waited more than four to five weeks for their replacement. There seemed to be an inexhaustible supply of donor organs. By the time six months had passed, Sharon had accrued a waiting list of more than 150 children from all over the United States, and some of the cases even came from other countries for their transplant surgeries. She was performing transplant surgery on thirty to forty children a month, and her spirits were the highest they had ever been.

A child was never lost because of the lack of a donor organ, and her success rate was nearly 100 percent. All the medical news journals and the local newspapers got wind of her successes, and her notoriety became widely publicized. Even the foreign media touted her success along with that of TWMC. Everything she had ever wished for was now a reality. There remained, however, in the back of her mind a nagging, which she managed to keep suppressed.

One morning, while attending the transplant clinic, one of the residents on the service, Doctor William Sorensen, discussed the medical problems of a specific patient with Sharon.

"Doctor Dell, I am stumped with a problem concerning Linda Korn, a seven-year-old referred to me for an evaluation for a possible liver transplant."

"Tell me about it, please." "She was referred by her pediatrician for advancing liver failure, which started twelve months ago. Linda's past history is completely negative for any congenital or acquired hepatic diseases, yet her liver function tests are all severely abnormal."

"What about her immunization history?"

"It's all timely, and there has been no documented evidence of any reactions or illness following them."

"What are your findings on physical examination?"

"She appears chronically ill and she is below the standard for height and weight. The liver is enlarged, the spleen tip is palpable, and she is jaundiced. The blood tests confirm she is approaching an end-stage liver status. In my opinion, she should be considered for transplant liver surgery. My question is, what is the source of her liver disease?"

"Have all the tests for the more esoteric liver diseases been performed?"

"Yes, they have."

"Well, let's go and see Linda together, Doctor Sorensen," said Sharon, and they walked to the examination room. Entering the small, brightly decorated room, they were met by Linda sitting on the floor holding a doll. Her mother was seated and appeared very anxious. Linda had blue eyes that were accentuated by the deeply pronounced yellow jaundice, which replaced the normal white sclera. Her long blonde hair fell almost to her waist. Linda hardly noticed them as she continued to talk to her doll. The exam rooms in Sharon's clinic were all created with the child in mind. All the walls were decorated with cartoon heroes as well as those of the latest fad. Some rooms were predominated by the Power Rangers, while others were inscribed with the Ninja Turtles, Batman, Superman, and many others. It was Sharon's intent that the children be put at ease while in her department so they would gain confidence in their doctors by transferring their acceptance of the surroundings. It was also required that all professional and non-professional personnel wear informal clothing, for the same purpose.

"Mrs. Korn, this is Dr. Dell, the Chief of Pediatric Transplant Surgery," said Doctor Sorensen, with a very apparent note of pride in his voice.

"How do you do, Mrs. Korn? I am happy to meet you. Doctor Sorensen and I have discussed Linda's condition, and there are a few questions I would like to ask you about it."

"Certainly, Doctor. What do you wish to know?"

"Mrs. Korn, did Linda have normal growth and development throughout her childhood?"

"Well yes, she did, until she had the operation on her right arm."

Hearing the response provoked an anxious question by Doctor Sorensen. "Mrs. Korn, you didn't tell me anything about an operation!"

"I'm sorry, Doctor, I guess I forgot about it."

Sharon moved toward Linda, who was still playing with her doll. "Hi sweetie, what's your dolly's name?" Within a few short minutes, Linda was completely at ease with Sharon, who was already examining the little girl. She focused her inspection on Linda's right arm, and only after looking very closely was she able to detect the scar at the shoulder level, which disappeared in the armpit.

"Tell me, what was this operation done for?"

"Linda was in an auto accident when she was four years old. She almost lost her arm because of multiple fractures. The doctors told us her blood and nerve supply to the arm was interrupted and she might lose her arm. She was in the hospital for two months and had three operations to save it."

"That's amazing. I'm delighted the outcome was successful. Did she have problems during her hospitalization, such as shock?"

"I don't think so."

"Did Linda receive any medications when she went home, such as antibiotics?"

"She did take antibiotics for about two weeks, as well as some other medication to help the healing process."

"How long did she take that medication?"

"Oh, she just stopped that one four or five months ago."

"Do you know the name of it?"

"No, I don't—the bottle only had a number on it along with Linda's name."

"Who prescribed it for you?"

"That's easy. It was Doctor Barry Swenz."

"And where is he located?"

"Why, right here, Doctor—in the Department of Pediatric Orthopedics."

Sharon was stunned. It was impossible to know all the doctors on the staff, but why hadn't that medical record accompanied Linda today? She was a bit perturbed about this and made a mental note to find out the answer. It would have been a simple task for the resident to review an existing medical record if it had been sent to the transplant clinic like it was supposed to be. She turned to Doctor Sorensen and said, "Linda needs to be admitted for a needle biopsy of the liver. Please make all the arrangements and explain the procedure to Mrs. Korn."

She turned to the mother. "Mrs. Korn, Doctor Sorensen will explain in detail what is needed. We would like to take a tiny piece of liver tissue for study in order to see if we can identify what caused this liver disease. After we do that, I'll talk to you about the next step."

Doctor Sorensen took his cue and began to explain the procedure in detail as Sharon left the room. She headed for her office with one thing in mind—she wanted to access Linda's medical record from her computer. Closing the door,

Sharon said to Shelly, her secretary, "I will be busy for about an hour. Please hold all my calls unless they are emergencies.

She accessed Linda Korn's medical record and read the index file that noted all admissions and outpatient visits chronologically. "There must be an error," she said to herself, shaking her head slowly from side to side. She then pulled up each clinic visit and perused the record. Nowhere in the record was there any mention of medication ordered by Doctor Swenz. After satisfying herself that the medical information was indeed that of her patient, she brought up the hospital patient files. There she found that Linda had been in the hospital for sixty-one days and had undergone two extensive surgical procedures on her right arm. Linda had sustained a traumatic amputation of her right arm slightly below the shoulder. The first operation for reattachment of the blood vessels and nerves had met with failure. Four weeks after the operation, the arm showed signs of nerve interruption, and a second operation was performed. According to the chart, the second procedure was successful, and after beginning a course of physical therapy, Linda was discharged home with the therapy program to continue at home twice weekly. Doctor Swenz in the pediatric orthopedic clinic then followed her until six months ago. There was something wrong with the record, but Sharon couldn't put her finger on it. She sat back in her chair and started to write out the salient medical facts when it hit her all at once. Where was the third surgery Mrs. Korn had told her about? There was no way a mother would not recall the correct number of surgeries on her child. She again went to the computer and tried to access other possible misfiled records by not only using the patient's name but also the medical record number, or even inputting the surgery type. The exercise proved fruitless. Sharon picked up her phone.

"Shelly, please call Medical Records and see if there are any other surgical records on Linda Korn besides the ones that are on the computer. Also, call Mrs. Korn and verify that there were three surgeries performed, please."

"Certainly Doctor Dell, anything else?"

"If you run up against a wall, perhaps you can find out something from Pediatric Orthopedics."

The following morning, Shelly approached Sharon.

"Doctor Dell, I confirmed with Mrs. Korn that three surgeries were performed on Linda during the same hospitalization. I ran up against a brick wall with Medical Records, and Ortho told me they didn't know anything since they don't keep past medical records in their department. Everything is supposed to be on the computer."

Sharon stared silently. *I've got to get to the bottom of this dilemma*, she thought to herself.

"Would you call Doctor Swenz and ask him if I can meet with him today, please?"

"Certainly, I'll call him right away."

Sharon returned to the heap of paperwork on her desk. A few moments later, Shelly called to tell her she had set up a meeting in Doctor Swenz's office at eleven o'clock. Sharon nodded and resumed her work. She hated this part of her job and usually procrastinated doing paperwork until the very last minute. At last, the appointed hour was upon her, and she headed for the Pediatric Orthopedics Department. She was greeted by the department secretary, who led her into Doctor Swenz's office.

Doctor Barry Swenz was very tall, about two hundred pounds, with a kindly face. He had dark brown eyes and wore an insincere smile while speaking.

"Doctor Dell, please sit down. I am very happy to meet you at last. As you probably know, I have been away on vacation over the last four weeks and have just returned to work recently. I apologize for not having formally introduced myself to you before this." We are isolated from the main hospital here, and I don't get over there much."

"Please don't apologize, Doctor Swenz. I realize how busy you must have been since your return to the hospital."

"To tell you the truth, Sharon—is it permissible to call you that?—it's been a zoo."

"Please do."

"Great then, please call me Barry."

"Alright." She was trying to get to the point of the meeting but was having difficulty in doing so because Doctor Swenz kept talking about her and she was unable to change the subject.

"How long have you been here, Sharon?"

"I have been here almost a year now, and it's been great."

"I've been apprised of your success and am delighted for you."

"I certainly don't foresee any moves in the near future. I've been happier here than I have been anywhere." "Well, I'm glad to hear you are not bored at our hospital. I hope you remain with us for a very long time."

"I'm doing a minimum of two transplants a day, and the most amazing thing about it is I have never lost a patient due to the unavailability of a donor organ."

"That's great. You must feel very good about being able to help so many children."

"I do. It's the fulfillment of a dream."

"Well tell me, Sharon, what did you want to see me about?"

"I want to speak to you about a mutual patient."

"Who is that?"

"Linda Korn. You operated on her right arm for a traumatic amputation about three years ago."

Swenz became slightly flushed as he cleared his throat. "I recall her case. What do you want to discuss?"

"I saw Linda in clinic a few days ago to evaluate her for a liver transplant. Her pediatrician, who had been documenting progressive liver failure for a period of months, referred her. Mrs. Korn told me about three operations that Linda had undergone. The patient's hospital chart did not accompany her to the clinic for some unknown reason, so I pulled it up on the computer and was only able to find two surgeries performed for the arm, not three."

"There were only two done. Mrs. Korn is obviously mistaken."

Sharon bit her lower lip when she heard Barry's answer. She knew Linda's mother could not have mistaken the total number of surgeries done on her daughter.

"Well, if that's all you want to know, Sharon, I am already late for a meeting. Please don't hesitate to call me anytime," said Doctor Swenz as he rose from his chair and started for the door with Sharon at his side. She was astounded at the abrupt manner in which Barry had brought the meeting to an end. It wasn't anything like the start of their discussion, which had led her to believe that the doctor had nothing to do and all day to do it in. She smiled pleasantly and left his office. *He acts as if he is trying to conceal something,* she thought as she waited for the elevator door to open.

$-4-$

THE CONSORTIUM

As soon as Sharon entered the elevator, Barry Swenz returned to his office and closed the door. He asked his secretary to hold all calls. He quickly dialed the CEO of TWMC.

"Doctor Swenz here, may I speak with Mr. Foxworthy, please?"

"Certainly Doctor, I'll tell him you're on the line."

"Hello Barry, how are you today?" asked James Foxworthy.

"I could be a whole lot better. We have a serious problem."

"I'm listening."

"I was just visited by Doctor Sharon Dell, the pediatric transplant surgeon. She questioned me about the Linda Korn case I did a few years ago. Remember?"

"Of course I remember. That was the first one we tested the KZ67 on. We had a hell of a time convincing our board to approve it."

"That's history, Jim. We now have a crisis on our hands, and I need your help. Doctor Dell has discovered that Linda had three surgeries and the medical records only reflect the fact she had two. She is snooping around, trying to dig up information. We have to stop her."

"Listen Barry, in view of the gravity of this development, I will ask our board of directors to convene an emergency meeting tomorrow night to consider alternatives."

"Fine. Let me know the time and place," said Barry as he slammed down the phone.

James Foxworthy hung up and buzzed his secretary. "Ann, call all the members of the board of directors and see if you can set up a meeting for tomorrow early evening. Tell them that this is an emergency, and see if the medical staff committee room on the seventh floor of the hospital will be available for the meeting."

"I'll get on it immediately," she answered smartly.

"Thank you, Ann. Let Doctor Swenz know when you have it set up."

"Certainly, Mr. Foxworthy."

Foxworthy sat back in his oversized plush desk chair and put his feet up on his elegant rosewood desk. As he shut his eyes, he started to perceive the migraine headache. The lighted office would only serve to accentuate the pain beginning over the right frontal area, but if he kept his eyes closed and concentrated on other things, the pain would often dissipate. Over the years, he'd grown to recognize that his migraines were the result of anxiety. If he was quick enough, the pain would soon be aborted, but sometimes when the pain became intense, it caused vomiting. It was his luck that Imitrex, the new wonder drug for migraine, was not effective at all for him. His mind wandered as he thought about the events that had led up to the recent crisis. It had been about three years ago when the TWMC Board gave approval for the use of the experimental drug KZ67, which had been developed by the Bently Drug Company. This was supposed to be the new wonder drug to prevent organ rejection. TWMC was desperately in need of a new anti-rejection drug because of the increasing number of rejections and deaths suffered by their post-transplant patients. Bently Drug Company was the leader in anti-rejection drug research and development, and it had risen to become a multibillion-dollar company. They had made a secret deal, giving ten million dollars yearly to the TWMC Board in return for supplying patients for their new drug research program. In reality, the company was buying human guinea pigs for new drug testing using non-FDA-approved drugs.

Promptly at 7 p.m., the board of directors of TWMC was called to order. Seated around the huge oval rosewood table were the seven members of the board. The oldest member was Alfred Russel, M.D., a man who appeared younger than his seventy years. He was slightly over six feet with thick salt-and-pepper wavy hair, wore bifocals, and spoke with a soft, gentle voice that complemented his demeanor. He was independently wealthy and was enjoying his retirement.

To his right sat James Foxworthy, a man of medium build, five feet eleven with sandy brown hair. His mannerisms were precise and deliberate, and he exuded an aura of extreme confidence and trust. With these qualities, he found it quite easy to endear himself to the physicians at TWMC and, as a result, was a very successful CEO. Physicians were a very difficult group to manage and get along with. Most of them thought they were experts in everything, including hospital administration, and it took the cunning and perseverance of this man to cultivate the physician leaders. Foxworthy had learned years before to weed the leaders out and to develop close ties with them. In this manner, he was able to get almost anything accomplished at the medical staff level, because doctors could be bought easily. They were a greedy lot who always responded to the offer of the green stuff. It amazed James how easy it was to buy political support for so little money. Just an offer to foot the bill for a week in Hawaii for two made to the right doctor was all it took to rope in the younger ones. The senior doctors, however, were much more demanding. It was worth it in the end, because James was able to get the medical staff's support for anything he wanted to do. This relationship with an unwieldy group of 150 physicians, each with their own agenda, was envied and respected by all the board members who had elected him as chairman.

Next to Foxworthy sat Doctor Barry Swenz, Chairman of the Department of Pediatric Orthopedics. He was forty-eight years old, had a thin build, and stood six feet two inches tall. He had an odd resemblance to Ichabod Crane when he walked. His arms and legs seemed to be all over the place. His arms swung far in front of his body and his stride tried in vain to keep pace with them. He wore his dark brown hair closely cropped.

Seated in the next chair was Michael Rome, President and Chairman of the Board of the Genome Corporation. This corporation was involved in the development of newer aspects of genetic engineering and was at the forefront of exciting new discoveries. Mr. David Malkin, the President and Chairman of the Board of Bently Drug Company, sat in the next chair, and on his other side was Seymour Kramer, President and Chairman of the Board of World Health Care, the largest HMO in the United States, with footholds in Europe and some smaller countries as well. Finally, next to him sat Mr. Richard Morris, an extremely wealthy gentleman, who rumor had it, was worth close to a billion dollars.

"Gentlemen, thank you all for being here on such short notice," said James Foxworthy. "We have very urgent business to discuss, so I will now turn the meeting over to Doctor Swenz." "Thank you, James. Gentlemen, I was paid a visit yesterday by Doctor Sharon Dell, Chief of the Department of Pediatric Transplant Surgery. She was attempting to find information about a surgery that I performed three years ago on Linda Korn. It seems Linda was referred to her to be evaluated for a liver transplant because of progressive liver failure. Due to a clerical error, no medical records appeared at the clinic, and Doctor Dell had to research them through the hospital's computer system. She found that Linda had undergone two operations on her right arm, but Mrs. Korn told her there were three operations performed during that hospitalization. Doctor Dell was not swayed by me when I assured her that Mrs. Korn was in error. I truly believe we haven't seen the end of her concerning this matter."

"Doctor Swenz," interrupted David Malkin," "is that the girl we tried the KZ67 on for the first time?"

"Yes it is, Dave. If you recall, Linda had sustained a

traumatic amputation to her right arm, which I repaired. Three weeks or so later, she developed evidence of neurological and vascular incompetence which necessitated the second operation. It was after the failure of the second surgery that we had the Board meeting, at which the use of the KZ67 in Linda was approved. The agreement was made between TWMC and Bently Drugs for financial support of our center. I followed her in the clinic until five months ago when I finally stopped the drug. I made entries in her clinic chart without mentioning anything specific about KZ67. At that time there was just a hint of liver enzyme elevation, but since then she has sustained further liver damage."

"Are you saying that the drug has caused liver toxicity and now she needs a liver?"

"I'm afraid I am." At that moment, the room became silent. The board members looked at each other and some shook their heads.

"That drug was given to Linda to help suppress her immune system after the third surgery, which was necessary to save her arm."

"Excuse me, if I may get a word in edgewise please," said Michael Rome. "If memory serves me correct, Genome provided the arm for Linda because she was losing hers, correct?"

"Yes, that's right," said Doctor Swenz. "She was the first patient to ever receive a genetically engineered extremity, which was developed at our research center, and the drug was given to prevent rejection from occurring. As you are all aware, whenever we do that type of surgical procedure, the medical records are kept under lock and key for obvious reasons. If anyone ever found out about our research, clinical testing and surgery, we'd all be in trouble." Fine beads of sweat appeared on Swenz's forehead.

"But look at all the good we do," said Doctor Russell. "Furthermore, it won't be much longer until we all make fortunes from all these developments." The other members nodded in agreement.

"Look," said Swenz, "Doctor Dell is no dummy, and if she finds out we used Linda as a guinea pig to test an anti-rejection drug, even though we gave her a new arm, she will expose us. That drug caused liver toxicity, and now Linda needs a liver transplant."

"So what?" interjected Seymour Kaplan. "She is one of our patients, and we pay all the bills. In addition, we have the livers available, don't we?"

"That is no problem. Just tell us when you want it," answered Michael Rome.

"I need your suggestions on how to proceed with Doctor Dell, gentlemen."

The room became uncomfortably silent for what seemed an eternity. James Foxworthy broke the silence at last. "Do you feel Sharon would be amenable to this aspect of the clinical research if she were filled in on the entire project?"

"I know she loves her work and position at TWMC and is ecstatic about all the lives she saves, but I'm not confident she would remain here if she knew 'everything,'" answered Barry Swenz.

"Well then, Barry, do you think she might blow the whistle

on us or just leave quietly?" asked Richard Morris somewhat nervously.

"I can't say for sure, Richard. I just don't know."

Seymour Kramer was feeling his share of anxiety and just couldn't remain seated any longer. He pushed his chair away from the table and stood up. The others gave him their attention in expectation. He walked around the large room in deep thought, totally oblivious to the rest of the board, and then stopped suddenly. His antics resembled a person who had just remembered something he had forgotten at home and was now wanting to return home to retrieve it. He was somewhat embarrassed to find the entire board staring at him.

"James, how well off financially is Doctor Dell?"

"I don't believe she is wealthy, but no doubt she is comfortable with the $160,000 a year we pay her."

"Is it possible we should consider raising her salary to $200,000 and include a sizable bonus upon signing a new contract?" asked Seymour.

"Anything is possible, but if I had to venture a guess, I'd say Doctor Dell's ethics and moral fiber would preclude that possibility. It might even provoke her to blow the whistle on us."

"We must come up with a plan to quiet this all down quickly," said Michael Rome.

"You've got my vote on that," chimed in David Malkin.

"Perhaps we should all go home and give this deep thought over this next week and then discuss it again. We can do it over the phone, but now I vote for adjournment," said Richard Morris.

"If there are no objections to the motion, this meeting is adjourned," said Foxworthy.

Barry Swenz drove home thinking about the meeting. Since his divorce, he'd lived alone in a swanky community. He knew who he had to call. Entering his house, he headed for the phone and placed the call.

"Hello, this is Barry Swenz. I hope it's not too late for me to call."

"No, not at all. I haven't turned in for the evening yet. What can I do for you?"

"Something very important has come up. Can we meet for lunch tomorrow, around one?"

"That would be fine. Where shall we meet?"

"What about Bernie's Grill on Central Avenue?"

"That will be fine. I'll see you tomorrow."

Barry hung up the phone and wandered into the living room, where he mixed himself a stiff gin and tonic. He sat on the couch and put his feet on the ottoman, closing his eyes. He considered the dilemma and asked himself why this had to happen now. The research was almost completed, and he would soon be a multimillionaire. His mind wandered back in time five years before, to the beginning of the project. He'd been told by David Malkin, President of Bently Drug Company, that there was a golden opportunity to perform surgeries that had never been done before. There was a catch, however—the efficacy of the new anti-rejection drug also had to be tested.

Dave said the FDA was so slow that currently available wonder drugs could take more than five years before gaining approval. Bently Drug Company had joint-ventured with the Genome Corporation to research and develop anti-rejection drugs. They were also pioneers in genetic engineering, which led to the rapid discovery of the location of the genes that promoted specific organ development. With this knowledge, they were able to direct the production of specific organs at will. The manner in which this genetic engineering feat was accomplished remained a closely guarded secret.

▲ ▲ ▲

It appeared the world market demand for donor organs was in chaos. Europe, Asia and South America had been invaded by a virulent new strain of hepatitis virus. For some unknown reason this new virus struck children in epidemic proportions, which ended in fatality for 20 percent of those affected. In such cases, the only chance for survival was a liver transplant. Bently Drug Company had immediately begun research in an attempt to find a drug that would kill the virus.

The strain caused a chronic hepatitis that rapidly led to liver failure in many cases, requiring liver transplants for survival. Bently's research techniques necessitated the use of an entire affected liver, and thus they joined with the Genome Corporation in their venture. In this manner, the Genome Corporation retrieved the diseased liver at the time of the transplant and, in return, arranged for the clinical research of the new anti-rejection drug.

Most of the countries involved in the epidemic had passed stringent laws about the disposal of the removed, hepatitis-infested livers. These livers were to be disposed of using stringent toxic waste procedures in order to prevent contamination. Genome started their own toxic waste disposal plants all over the world, but was very careful to pick up these livers at the time of the transplant and transport them to the various strategically situated Bently labs. The livers were fresh upon arrival, and immediate viral extraction procedures and scientific research were conducted.

The third partner in the joint venture was the large HMO World Health Care. They were hit hard financially by the hepatitis epidemic because of financial responsibility for the increased number of liver transplants. Their own economic statisticians predicted gloom unless the number of transplants were significantly reduced. However, it now looked like the number of transplants was on the rise. It was of financial benefit to the HMO to join the venture and contribute to the research and development of a drug to eradicate the virus. Of course, there was also a parallel effort to produce an antigen so the world could be inoculated prophylactically. These new drugs could prevent the HMO from financial disaster.

After all was said and done, the symbiotic relationship of these three financial giants would be an eventual boon to all of their bottom lines. An added plus from World Health Care was that they gave their permission for all their transplant patients at TWMC to be used in clinical research and drug evaluation. They reasoned that the more patients committed to this research, the quicker the drug cure for the virus would be found and the faster they would be able to stem their financial losses. The HMO was able to control the patient case review process for proper utilization, as well as for quality parameters, on all their patients by establishing a method to bypass standard medical reviews. This was extremely important—otherwise, some doctor reviewing the clinical chart might discover the patient was used in an unauthorized clinical drug research evaluation and create unnecessary problems. The Genome Corporation provided the genetically engineered livers for their cost while also harvesting the diseased livers for Bently's research. Bently provided the anti-rejection drug for the clinical trials and was also deeply involved in researching a drug to kill the virus, as well as one to prevent the hepatitis infection. World Health Care contributed patients for the study and millions of dollars to the project. The short-term gain from the joint venture during the experimental stage was measured in what they derived from each other. The long-term gain they were all acutely aware of was the billions of dollars they would share in at the completion of the research phase when their discoveries were marketed.

The lobbyists hired by each of the corporations predicted uniformly that once Europe had approved KZ67 and Genome's livers were for sale on the open market, the pressure levied upon the FDA would be intolerable and the FDA would be quick to grant their approval.

Bently Drug Company anticipated Europe's approval for KZ67 in short order. They all knew that once that occurred, it was only a matter of time before Genome Corporation leaked the news to the press that it had developed the genetic process by which organs could be developed. The European countries were reeling from the hepatitis epidemic and were ready and very willing to purchase organs for those children who required them. The money would come from both the private as well as the governmental sector. Political pressure would mandate that governments act quickly to purchase the livers, and where socialized medicine was not the impetus, private funding would be available throughout the European banking system. The World Bank had issued their written guarantee to these banking institutions to back all loans made to private citizens for these purchases. This, of course, became a strong stimulus in the economy of nations as well. It was obvious that the driving force for the joint venture of the three giants with TWMC was greed. The board of directors, after overcoming a minor obstacle with the chairman, was very willing to agree with the three companies to allow the clinical research, both drugs and surgery, to be done at TWMC for the sum of ten million dollars per year. Of course there was also a "signing bonus" of $150,000 a year, which would be paid to each of the board members as a consulting fee.

-5-

THE THIRD SURGERY

Bernie's Grill was located just outside the business district of the city of San Bernardino. Promptly at 1 p.m., Doctor Barry Swenz walked through the front door and was greeted by the maître d', who led him through the dining room crammed with mid-day diners to a small table located in a secluded corner. As he approached the table, an attractive blonde woman about thirty-five years old smiled and greeted him.

"I'm delighted to see you again, Doctor Swenz. It's been at least five months since we've spoken."

"It's good to see you also," responded Barry.

She was sipping a tall glass of iced tea as he sat down across from her. After exchanging the usual pleasantries, Barry looked at his watch.

"I don't have much time, Mrs. Korn, so I will cut to the chase. We have a slight problem that I must speak with you about."

"Certainly, what is it?"

"I'm sure you must have recognized during your daughter's visit with Doctor Dell that the doctor was very interested in finding out about the third operation."

"Yes, she caught me off guard. I told her three surgeries were done by a slip of the tongue. I know you told me to forget the third one. I'm really sorry."

As the waiter approached to take their orders, he signaled Ruth to remain silent. A few moments later, he continued on.

"If Doctor Dell discovers what we have done, we'll all be in big trouble. What's more important is that you won't receive any more money from TWMC."

Ruth Korn looked shocked. She thought about the three-thousand-dollar-a-month stipend she received from TWMC. She was carried on their payroll as an executive secretary for special services.

"What can I do?" she asked angrily.

"Nothing. I just want to alert you that there may be a problem in the future and to make you aware in case Doctor Dell asks you more questions."

They conversed for another twenty minutes, then Barry made his apologies for not staying longer, summoned the waiter, paid the check, and took his leave. Ruth sat in anxious silence. She closed her eyes and thought about the problem. Her mind focused on the first meeting with Doctor Swenz, years ago, when Linda had been hospitalized after her accident. After Linda's second surgery did not succeed in correcting the failure of the nerves and blood vessels to unite, Doctor Swenz asked her to come to his office to discuss Linda's case.

She confided in him then that Linda was not her daughter. She had been married to Gary for seven years and Gary had a daughter, Linda, from his previous short marriage. Linda's biological mother was committed for life to the Camarillo State Mental Hospital with the diagnosis of paranoid schizophrenia and after numerous suicidal as well as homicidal attempts. Because of all the attention Linda required, Gary felt neglected, and one day he walked out on the marriage never to be heard from again. Since Ruth and Linda had the same last name, she saw no need to petition the court for a formal adoption. Because of this fact, it wasn't ever a problem to sign all the necessary consents as her real mother.

Doctor Swenz explained that Linda was going to lose her arm because of the failure of the operations to restore neurovascular competence. Unbeknown to her, Doctor Swenz was awaiting just such a patient. The TWMC board of directors had not yet consented to allow clinical research to occur. They had met for initial discussions and felt somewhat intimidated by the proposal of the three large companies. Bently Drug Company had disclosed their 100-percent success rate with the anti-rejection drug KZ67 in primates, but it had never been tried in humans. The Genome Corporation had successfully developed the genetic engineering for production of extremities or limbs, but surgical transplantation had yet to be attempted in humans. It was this combination of events that led to the discussions with Swenz, as a noted pediatric orthopedic surgeon. He was promised the sum of twenty million dollars once these new products were approved for sale. The impetus was directed at the foreign market, where there was no foreseeable delay in obtaining drug approval. The companies convinced Swenz that once the products were available on the foreign market, the U.S. would soon follow. The political clout had already been put into motion by the corporations' lobbyists.

Linda Korn just happened to suffer her accident at the right time, and Doctor Swenz was convinced that if he were to restore her extremity without rejection, the board would have to agree to the proposal made by the joint venture companies. Genome and Bently also agreed to pay Swenz an additional $200,000 to perform the surgery and to manage the postoperative anti-rejection drug therapy. He was already convinced of the need for this clinical research in his own mind anyway, but the cash inducement forced him into quick action.

"Mrs. Korn, there is now available a genetically engineered arm that Genome has developed and experimented with for years. They feel they have a superior product and would like Linda to be the first patient to have it."

"Is it safe, Doctor?"

"She wouldn't be any worse off if she lost her arm today. If the new drug doesn't work, rejection is a certainty and she will lose the new arm also. We are offering her a new chance for an arm, but it must be kept secret."

"Why is that?"

"Because these procedures are not FDA approved as yet. They take years to approve new drugs and techniques such as a genetically engineered extremity."

"Linda would be the first human ever to have the arm or the drug?"

"That's true, but I urge you to consider the alternative. She would go through life with a mechanical prosthetic arm."

Ruth saw an opportunity now. She perceived that Doctor Swenz was pushing hard for her approval. He was very persuasive in his presentation, but it lacked the element of total objectivity. In his eagerness, he shied away from any of the dangers or negative aspects of the drug therapy. She had been witness to a friend who had undertaken chemotherapy and had seen the immense side effects. "Doctor Swenz, I might consent to this plan for therapy if the companies involved would pay Linda a sum of money yearly until she becomes eighteen years old. That would guarantee her ability to attend college. Of course, I would also insist upon a monthly allowance so that I might provide the necessities for her. I am on welfare, so I can be at home with Linda and her sister Sara, who was born with a genetic defect called Penta X syndrome. Sara is my daughter from a previous marriage." She explained that she was told that it was a genetic disorder that affected females only, with them inheriting three extra X chromosomes. Their body cells all had five X chromosomes as opposed to only two.

"I was unaware of that, Ruth. Please tell me about Sara's problems."

"It is a chromosomal defect that's resulted in Mongolism, enlarged heart and kidney failure. Sara underwent a kidney transplant six years ago at the age of five."

Doctor Swenz was amazed. This mother certainly had her hands full with two sick children, and she was now asking for financial help to weather the storms of life with some degree of financial certainty. He was deeply moved by her story, and his compassion was overwhelming.

"I will request that the hospital strongly consider your request."

"Thank you, Doctor Swenz. All I care about are these children. If you can convince the hospital to agree with my request, I'll consent immediately."

"I'll call you tomorrow and let you know their decision." He then ushered her out of his office. Linda was not privy to what happened next.

Barry returned to his desk and picked up the phone.

"Hello, this is Doctor Swenz, may I speak with Mr. Foxworthy?"

"Please hold, Doctor. I'll let him know you are on the line," replied the secretary.

A moment later, Jim Foxworthy was on the phone. "Doctor Swenz, how are you today?"

"Jim, I have almost convinced Mrs. Korn to consent to the genetic arm replacement for her daughter Linda, but at a cost. She is requesting a monthly stipend for both herself and her daughter." He conveyed the details of their conversation. "If it's a success, the hospital board will agree to the joint venture with Genome Corporation, Bently, and World Health Care. All we need is one successful surgery to convince them to forge ahead with the joint venture agreement. You know that the entire board must be in agreement to do this partnership. The key man necessary for the deal is Doctor Russell. His hangup is centered on the possibility of failure and complications. I have spoken with him about it, and he will agree to the venture if he sees a good result from the surgery.

"Let me speak with some of the board and get their

permission. If I get the green light, I can add her to our payroll without difficulty."

"Fine. Can you get back to me before tomorrow? I promised Mrs. Korn I would call her back by then."

"Sure can." Hanging up the phone, he buzzed his secretary.

Within three hours, Jim Foxworthy had obtained the consent he required to place Mrs. Korn on the payroll, and he notified Doctor Swenz. Swenz called Ruth and arranged for her to sign both the consent and the *employment contract* at Mr. Foxworthy's office the next morning.

– 6 –

MEDICAL DETECTIVE WORK

Sharon was at her desk completing paperwork when Doctor Sorensen entered the office. "Excuse me, Doctor Dell, but I have a pressing problem that requires your immediate attention," he said, sounding exasperated. In his hands he held laboratory reports and a patient's chart.

"What is it, Doctor?"

"Last week I examined an eight-year-old boy who was referred for the possibility of liver transplantation. He has been developing progressive liver failure for almost a year now. When I finished taking a meticulous history, I could not pinpoint the reason for the liver disease. I asked the standard questions regarding surgeries and accidents, looking for the possibility of hepatitis from blood transfusions. I was shocked to learn from the mother that her son Jason had been a patient here three years ago. You'll never guess what he was here for!"

"I can't imagine. Please tell me."

"He was struck by an automobile while on his tricycle. His injuries included crush wounds to the chest. He was DOA when he arrived here, but an aggressive ER Doctor did CPR and restored his cardiovascular collapse. I read the entire hospital chart and discovered that he underwent surgery for a cardiac rupture and received a heart transplant performed by Doctor Henry Walker, the Chief of Pediatric Cardiac Surgery."

"So far I don't see anything out of the ordinary," said Sharon.

"I'm coming to the best part now. The surgery took place within four weeks of admission, and Jason had been seeing Doctor Swenz in follow-up at Peds Ortho Clinic until a year ago when he was discharged from the clinic."

"What were the orthopedic problems all about?"

"That's just it, Doctor Dell—there really weren't any, except for the blunt trauma he received to his chest. There were no fractures and no other orthopedic problems listed anywhere in the chart!"

"Are you telling me that this child was followed in our Peds Ortho Clinic for two years without an orthopedic diagnosis?"

"Yes! There is an occasional mention about vague pains in the arms and back, but nothing else. Certainly nothing that would justify clinic visits every four weeks for two years."

"You must have overlooked something, Doctor," Sharon said with outstretched hands and raised eyebrows, suggesting disbelief.

"I thought that also, so after I reviewed the chart again, I called Mrs. Myrick and had a very interesting chat with her."

"Tell me!" said Sharon impatiently.

"Mrs. Myrick was told that Jason had to receive a drug to prevent rejection from occurring and that Doctor Swenz was an expert in that area. She received a new bottle of pills directly from Doctor Swenz at each visit. Although there is no written documentation of this, the usual blood tests were drawn each time to evaluate the possibility of rejection. All the blood tests during the two years were normal, and Jason was discharged from the clinic care. Her pediatrician told her about a year ago that Jason had a mild liver inflammation. He ran all the usual tests for hepatitis, as well as all the other esoteric studies, and was unable to come up with a diagnosis. The liver test results became worse, and recently all the enzymes have doubled in value, indicating worsening liver failure. Clinically this child looks like he will need a transplant within two to three months. Jason is now developing bleeding due to the low prothrombin."

Sharon sat wide-eyed in shock over what she had just heard. She had suspected Doctor Swenz was deeply involved with Linda Korn's third surgery, and now there was more evidence that pointed in the same direction.

"Leave the chart and the laboratory reports with me for now, Doctor Sorensen. Thank you for an excellent piece of detective work, and please keep this to yourself for now. After I review all the data, I will call you, and perhaps we can sort this all out together."

Sorensen beamed with pride. It wasn't every day that he received such compliments.

She sat back in her chair and began to focus on the issues

just presented to her. *Doctor Swenz was involved in the postoperative care of two children, each with a different surgical procedure and both with liver failure requiring a liver transplant. What's even more confusing is that Swenz followed Jason for two years and he's an orthopedist. It would make sense that a cardiology specialist would follow a postoperative heart transplant patient, not an orthopedist. And if that's not enough already, how do you explain the rapidity with which a cardiac donor was found for Jason?*

She opened the chart and read each page slowly, making notes as she went. When she finished, she picked up the phone and dialed Doctor Henry Walker's office.

"This is Doctor Dell in Pediatric Liver Transplant, may I speak with Doctor Walker?"

"Why certainly, Doctor, I'll put you right through," said the secretary.

"This is Henry Walkler speaking."

"Doctor Walkler, this is Sharon Dell. Do you have a moment to discuss a case with me?"

"Certainly Sharon, and please, call me Henry."

"Thank you, Henry. Do you recall a Jason Myrick you operated on about three years ago?"

"No, I can't say that I do."

"He sustained a ruptured heart as a result of being hit by a car while riding his tricycle."

"Oh, sure … Yes, I ah, remember that case now," he replied in a tone of uncertainty.

"Tell me Henry, if you can remember, how you got a heart donor so quickly. You had him in surgery about four weeks after he was admitted to the hospital. No one ever gets a donor heart until they have been on the waiting list for at least six months."

"To tell you the truth, I really don't recall the specifics of that case. It was three years ago. All I recall is that he did *very* well after the surgery," answered Henry with a note of superiority.

"That brings me to my next question. Why was his postoperative cardiac care assigned to Doctor Swenz the orthopedist?"

The phone remained silent for what seemed like an eternity, and finally Doctor Winkler answered.

"I believe Jason was an HMO patient. As I recall, it was World Care, and they have a contractual provider contract with Doctor Swenz, to whom they refer all of our cardiac transplant follow-ups for postoperative care."

Sharon raised her eyebrows in disbelief. "You mean Doctor Swenz cares for all your transplant patients?" "Yes, I'm afraid that is the way things are set up here. I am not in agreement with that protocol—however, I have nothing to say about it. Once I finish the surgery, I follow the patient in the hospital, but all the anti-rejection drugs are ordered by Swenz. The HMO dictates this."

"What about the possibility of cardiac complications such as congestive heart failure or cardiac arrhythmias? An orthopod can't handle those!"

"Absolutely. I couldn't agree with you more, and as a matter of fact, Doctor Swenz allows one of my staff to examine our patients after he finishes up with them at each clinic visit. In that manner, we keep tabs on each patient in our own chart that we keep here in the department."

"Well at least the patients are getting proper follow-up medical care by the appropriate specialist. Thank you for your time, Henry." She hung up the phone and closed her eyes, resting her elbows on the desk. *This is very strange,* she thought. *I wonder what the protocol is with Doctor Moss's patients.*

Quickly, she dialed Garry Moss's telephone number.

"Hello Doctor Dell, how are you today?"

"Fine, Doctor Moss. I would like to ask you a question or two, if you have a moment?"

"Fire away. I've got to be in surgery in a few minutes."

"Who manages your patients' postoperative care?

"Why, we do."

"Do you regulate the anti-rejection drug therapy?"

"Ah ... well, no, we sort of do it in conjunction with Doctor Swenz, and other times it is done by our renal doctors exclusively."

"What determines which patients are referred to Doctor Swenz for follow-up care versus your own department doctors?"

"That's an easy one—all the HMO patients are referred to Swenz, and all the other ones we take care of. Our doctors also see the patients that Doctor Swenz sees in clinic on the same day. We maintain our own patient charts for each case."

"Tell me Doctor, have you noticed any instances of liver failure in your patients?"

"That's an interesting question. We have seen a number of liver failure patients that we referred for transplant surgery."

"What was the cause of the liver disease?"

"We never have found out. All those cases were referred to Squire Hospital in San Diego for transplant surgery."

"I don't understand. Why were they referred there?"

"That's where we were instructed to refer them by the HMO. Evidently they have a contract for liver transplant surgery at Squire."

"Wait a minute. Are you telling me that all of your patients who needed a liver transplant were referred to Squire Hospital?"

"Yes."

"How many patients were there?"

"I think about six or so."

"Were they all HMO patients, or were some of them from other health plans?"

"Interesting question. I never thought about it before. Now that you bring it up, I believe all the patients that needed liver transplants were HMO patients."

"Were any of the patients post-transplant?"

"Why, yes. As a matter of fact, they all had undergone either kidney or liver transplants."

Sharon held the phone and was too stunned to speak. Finally, she thanked Doctor Moss and hung up. She was confused and scared. What was going on? How could it be possible that only patients who belonged to the HMO came down with terminal liver disease requiring a transplant? There had to be a common denominator. Not only were kidney patients at risk for developing liver failure, but also kidney and heart transplant patients as well. But how did Linda Korn fit into the scenario? She'd only had surgery on her upper extremity.

Wait a minute! I was never able to find out the nature of her third surgery.

Sharon realized there had to be a link between Linda's liver failure and that of the other transplant patients. The patients of Doctor Moss had all been referred to another hospital for their liver transplants. Why had they not been referred to her or Doctor Moss for the transplant? Something was very wrong. *It's a good thing I'm leaving for the Olympics in Atlanta,* she thought.

Sharon knew she had to stop thinking about all she had discovered. She needed to clear her mind. Leaving TWMC, she drove home to pack. She was booked on the Delta noon flight leaving Los Angeles International Airport the next day.

— 7 —

UNSUCCESSFUL ATTEMPT

The jumbo jet taxied to the runway and revved the engines. A moment later, Sharon was asleep as the plane's engines strained at full throttle to gain altitude. She was emotionally drained and fatigued, brought about by the recent week's events at the hospital. In the pit of her stomach, she knew something was very wrong within the confines of TWMC, but despite her efforts, she had been unable to sort out the dilemma.

She had spoken with her colleagues and was convinced there was some kind of coverup going on within the hospital. A few days ago she had called World Health Care and, after the many transfers and voicemail commands, finally spoken with the Medical Director. He had been somewhat evasive regarding the pointed questions concerning Doctor Swenz's ability to properly care for postoperative transplant patients who were beyond his area of expertise. The Medical Director assured Sharon that the patients were all receiving the proper care as far as he knew. When she asked him if he was cognizant of the increased incidence of liver failure in the transplant patients, he became silent and then stuttered a bit, which indicated to Sharon that he was very much aware. He also avoided answering her question as to why those patients were all being referred to Squire Hospital in San Diego for the transplant surgery, mentioning something about better contracting rates.

She was suddenly awakened by the flight attendant asking her to fasten her seatbelt for landing. Within ten minutes, Sharon was walking through the massive Delta terminal to get her baggage. Claiming her two pieces of luggage, she headed to the Avis Car Rental booth and picked up her awaiting compact. She was familiar with Atlanta since one of her closest girlfriends had moved there years ago and Sharon had visited her from time to time. Leaving the airport, she headed south to Interstate 285 and then on to US 85, which led directly to US 75. Sharon considered herself fortunate to have secured accommodations only twelve miles from Atlanta. She drove off the interstate at Exit 73 and found her motel. The American Inn had just opened for business in time for the Olympics. She checked in, then went to her room, where she changed into shorts and a cool green cotton blouse that served to complement her complexion and accent her hazel eyes. Her light brown long hair was placed in a ponytail, and in her colorful Nikes, she looked as though she were a teenager. After driving to a local steak house, she returned to get an early night's rest. The track and field events were being held at the Olympic Stadium at 8:30 in the morning, which meant that she had to be up at 6:00. After hearing the traffic report on WGST she opted to ride the MARTA. She parked her car in the designated lot located only a few miles away in the town of Morro and boarded the bus at seven. She was deposited half a mile from the Olympic stadium gates. The security of the stadium mandated that a half-mile circumference of safety be provided, which made for a nice morning walk. At the stadium gates were positioned a series of ten metal detectors with adjacent tables. The lines, though very long, moved with ease as security personnel examined all portable objects, from cameras to lunch bags. The mood of the crowd was congenial and the accents were diverse. People wearing baseball caps designed with national flags and speaking in their native tongues gave the atmosphere of being in a foreign country. Some of the crowd were waving flags while t-shirt vendors hawked their wares and others offered cold drinks from their medium-sized Igloo cold boxes. Unknown to most of the eager crowd, the prices for the refreshments outside were cheap compared to the prices inside the gates. It only took one time for most people to discover this before they resorted to packing their own lunches, dinners, and drinks. They refused to be victims of the insane prices and restricted selection within the stadium gates.

Sharon sat through the morning session of the track and field events in awe of the athletic prowess she felt privileged to witness. At 1 p.m., she left the stadium and made her way amid the throngs of humanity to the designated MARTA station, where she was transported back to the lot in Morro. Getting out the map, she ascertained the most direct route to Conyers, where the equestrian venue was located. The Jumping events were scheduled to begin at 2:30 and she was fortunate enough to have tickets. She drove along Georgia's Route 138 and on to the venue site, where she exited at a sign indicating church parking for the equestrian event. She was directed off the road for about a half-mile and onto a large field in back of the church. No one was collecting money so she drove on, following the dirt road to the end where a few cars were parked. The field was very isolated and overlooked the designated parking area for the Atlanta Committee of Games (ACOG) building. In order to get to the bus that transported patrons ten miles to the venue, she had to walk along a narrow dirt path for a quarter mile which bisected a dense tangle of trees and undergrowth. She parked her car and opened the door just in time to be met by a thunderstorm. The thunder scared her in its abruptness as the heavens opened up with torrential rains. She unfolded her umbrella and the drops beat upon its shield while the thunder and lightning played out their supporting roles.

The midsize dark sedan had stayed close behind Sharon all the way from the MARTA lot in Morro. The sinister-looking man driving was thirty-five years old and a drug addict. When he had been approached for this job, he'd gladly accepted. Five thousand dollars and expenses to Atlanta were a dream come true for Randy Stone. He was on parole in California for aggravated assault and attempted murder and had just served seven years in the State Penitentiary at Chino. This was a down-and-dirty quickie deal which would get him home in three days before anyone would know he was gone. All he had to do was see that the good Doctor Dell met with an unfortunate deadly accident. When he saw that she was pulling into the large field leading up to the dense wooded area, he rapidly veered off the road and sped to the far end of the field, where he turned right and raced down the dirt road to the woods. He could still see her car about a half-mile to his left as it approached the end of the field that abutted the woods. After parking quickly, he ran from his car into the woods toward the field. He was hoping that she would have to walk through the woods on the dirt trail that led from the field. The woods were very dark, as the trees blocked most of the light. He was out of breath running through the dense trees and underbrush when he finally reached within twenty feet of the trail.

Randy was in luck. No one was about, except for Sharon, as she made her way along the trail in the midst of the storm. The rain had caused the path to become muddy with the red earth, and rivulets of water ran down as it sloped toward the designated parking lot. He buried himself in the dense underbrush about ten feet from the trail. Sharon was within twenty feet of the waiting assailant when thunder sounded as though it were a bomb. Randy pulled the nylon mask over his face and leaped at Sharon as she passed him. He lunged out and grabbed her around the neck, throwing her to the ground. She screamed in terror as he placed his hands around her throat, but they were slippery because of the rain. She managed to hold on to her umbrella and looped the handle around his neck from behind while he straddled her. Caught by surprise, he turned his head and she pulled with all her strength, which threw him off balance.

As he rolled to the side, the handle became free. Sharon was on her feet in a microsecond and quickly grabbed the handle of the umbrella. Randy rose from his knees to face her and was met with a violent stab in the groin. He doubled up in pain as a wave of nausea came over him and he fell to his knees. Sharon gripped the umbrella by the tip and with all the strength she could muster swung it down upon her assailant's head, breaking the handle. Randy's scalp split open along the hair line as he fell forward into the mud. She ran along the path as fast as she could to the parking lot, screaming at the top of her voice for help.

A mounted policeman patrolling the ACOG lot heard her cry and galloped toward her. Rapidly, she told him of the attack and he galloped off in the direction she indicated with his service revolver in his hand. Sharon sat down on the wet grass. She was shaking all over. *Why would anyone want to kill me? I don't know anyone here except my girlfriend!*

–8–

THE RESEARCH LABORATORY

The research facilities of Genome Corporation and Bently Drug Company were located in a three-story building that sprawled over a hundred-acre estate hidden within the confines of the Malibu Mountains. The 100,000-square-foot facility was surrounded by a ten-foot-high chain-link fence with razor wire coiled at the top. A short private road was the only approach to the building. A guard maintained security at the private road entrance from a twelve-foot tower, and other towers followed the fence line. State-of-the-art security devices protected the facility from intruders. Motion detectors, heat detectors, and video cameras were installed at strategic points along the fence's perimeter. Security clearance to gain entrance to the building was limited to those who worked for the companies. A special clearance beyond that was required to gain access to the third floor of the building. All visitors who had business with the facility were escorted to and from their appointments. It was known that the first floor housed and cared for the research animals, while all the actual re-search was carried out on the second floor. The third floor housed a closely guarded secret, and only four people had access to it. All stairway accesses and doors were secured by both voice and fingerprint codes.

The four who had free access to the third floor were Michael Rome, CEO and Chairman of the Board for the Genome Corporation, David Malkin, CEO and Chairman of the Board of Bently Drug Company, Doctor Paul Cook, Chief of Genome's research department, and Doctor Victor Matson, Chief of Bently's Drug Company Research Department.

Doctor Cook had received his MD and Ph.D. from Harvard University. He was board certified in obstetrics and gynecology, and his Ph.D. was in genetics. His specialty area was genetic mapping. Doctor Matson was also an MD and Ph.D. He was board certified in internal medicine and infec-tious diseases. He had recently stepped down from the pres-tigious CDC, where he had been the director of the Virology Department. He'd received his Ph.D in Pharmacology at the University of Chicago. Both doctors had published exten-sively in medical and scientific journals. Because of their im-mense stature, they were paid exceedingly well and were on a first-name basis with their CEOs. When the joint venture oc-curred, the CEOs met with each of these doctors and worked out certain bonuses to their satisfaction. Rome and Malkin both knew it would be prudent to certify the fidelity of the doctors, and they also knew that each man had his price. An ingenious plan to receive tax-free dollars was agreed upon by everyone. Each company agreed to set aside funds that were to be used exclusively to fund the college education of the children of both Doctors Matson and Cook. This was no paltry sum, since they each had four children and it was a sure bet that they would all go to college. Since both companies had already set aside modest sums of money for their employees to further their education, it was an easy task for them to perform. In this manner, all the children would be guaranteed a minimum of four years of college education with tuition, books, and all reasonable living expenses. This was written off as an expense by the companies, and the doctors would not have to pay taxes on the funds. When the kids drew the funds, they would pay taxes in their brackets which were substantially lower than their father's. The physicians calculated this was worth a minimum of thirty thousand dollars per year per child, or almost a half-million dollars for their children's education. Because the written agreements were to be kept private, no suspicion would be raised by an audit, should one occur.

Doctors Cook and Matson were having their weekly meeting at the Research Laboratories, a necessity in order to update each other in their respective research progress. They met in the conference room, which was soundproofed. There had always existed some element of jealousy between the researchers as was typical in the profession. Breakthroughs were happening frequently and it was imperative that they were kept informed of each other's advances. Many times, new discoveries would lead to a shortcut procedure in one of their labs.

"We are making a lot of headway with the hepatitis vaccine," said Matson eagerly.

"How long before you will have an antigen we can test?" asked Cook.

"I'm not certain, but I would estimate about another month or two," answered Matson.

"On another note, I received a call from Michael Rome, who has been in touch with Barry Swenz about a potential problem, and he asked me to discuss it with you to see if we can suggest a plan. He wants us to meet with him after you and I talk," said Matson with a very serious demeanor.

"Alright, let's discuss it now while I have the time," answered Cook, slightly annoyed with his colleague.

"It seems that a transplant surgeon at TWMC has been asking a lot of questions about the Linda Korn case. Her name is Doctor Sharon Dell."

"That was the first experimental patient that received a genetically engineered extremity," interjected Cook.

"Yes, and if you recall, we started her on KZ67, the anti-rejection drug as well."

"KZ67 has been working well, hasn't it?"

"As I now have been told, it seems there has been a slight problem," said Matson, raising his eyebrows while sighing deeply. "The drug seems to cause a delayed type of hepatitis. The liver injury has become chronic and now has led to the need for a liver transplant."

"My God! Why haven't we been informed until now?"

"From what I gather, there have been about a half-dozen such cases to date, and all but one was referred to Squire

Hospital in San Diego for the transplant to avoid any possibility of negative publicity. Linda Korn slipped into TWMC, and when Doctor Dell became aware that she'd had a third surgery on her traumatically amputated arm without any hospital records to verify it, she began asking a lot of questions. Doctor Barry Swenz, who has been following Linda's case, is very anxious about it, and with good reason."

"And we are supposed to figure out a way to coax Doctor Dell to join us in our endeavors?" asked Cook.

"Yes. Did Mike Rome tell you why we were never informed of the other cases before now?" asked Matson heatedly.

"He said there was only presumptive evidence and since there were only a few cases, the decision was to wait and observe. The diseased livers were examined by the hospital pathologist and diagnosed with viral hepatitis as the cause, at least from a histological point of view. None of the standard viral blood tests were positive, and since the new strain endemic in Europe had appeared, they were content to sign it out as atypical hepatitis."

"I assume all those cases had received organs other than livers?" asked Matson.

"There were three kidney transplants, one heart, one liver, and an extremity."

"Have you reviewed any of the medical records?" asked Matson.

"I looked at them briefly and strongly suspect that the hepatitis could have been prevented if steroids had been continued for at least a year after the KZ67 was terminated."

Matson shook his head slowly. He was visibly shaken with this news. He sat up straight in his chair and spoke. "I think we should get back to the problem at hand; we can review all the clinical data in the patient charts later. What is Barry Swenz's opinion concerning Doctor Dell?"

"From what I gather, she is a very dedicated doctor. She is very ethical and extremely altruistic."

"Has anyone tried to broach the subject with her?" inquired Matson impatiently.

"Mike told me that it was the opinion of the TWMC Board of Directors that we should try to develop a plan and then get back to him. He will pass it on to the board."

"Has anyone spoken to any of her colleagues or friends who really know her?" asked Cook hesitantly.

"That's a very good question, Paul. I don't think so."

"Perhaps it would be the better part of valor to seriously investigate Doctor Dell so we know her psyche, and then we might be able to devise a plan."

"Good idea! I will call Mike Rome and suggest that someone compile a dossier on her, and then we will discuss her."

"Fine then, I'll await your call." Matson stood up and walked to the door while Paul Cook was dialing Mike Rome's number. When he had finished, he hung up the phone and sighed deeply.

James Foxworthy was listening intently to Mike Rome's summary of what was needed. Foxworthy promised him he would hire a private detective to gather all possible information on Sharon Dell rapidly. As soon as he had the dossier, he would notify Rome. He made his call and hired a local private detective firm for the task. After agreeing to pay five thousand dollars, he was assured that the report would be on his desk in one week.

– 9 –

THE DOSSIER

Sharon had returned from the Olympics and was still very anxious over the attempt on her life. The police had not arrested anyone, and the event had been related to the San Bernardino Sheriff's Department by the Atlanta Police. She was contacted by the department and had answered all of their questions in an exhausting two-hour session the day after her return home. They had told her to keep in contact with them and to call if she had any suspicions about anyone. She agreed to do so, but she couldn't come up with any ideas at the moment. It was time to call her father and get his advice and consolation. That evening, she called Doctor Dell in Auburn and was relieved to find him at home.

"Hi Dad, how are you? I missed you. I just got back from the Olympics yesterday. I'll be returning to work tomorrow."

"Did you enjoy yourself, Sharon?"

There was a prolonged silence, which Karl quickly identified as a problem with his question. "What is it Sharon? I can tell you are upset about something."

"You always could, so why am I surprised that you picked

that up now," she said with a nervous laugh. "Well, it's not a pretty story, so sit down and I'll fill you in."

"I'm sitting."

"One day I went to the equestrian center in Conyers outside of Atlanta and had a big problem. I parked some distance from the shuttle pick-up point. I arrived just in time to be caught in a severe thunderstorm. I had to walk along a dirt trail that led through a patch of dense forest in order to get to the shuttle area, which was near the public parking lot. I would guess it was about a half-mile away. I arrived late, so no one was around when I parked in the church meadow nearby. When I started down the trail, the storm began and buckets of water fell from the sky. Within minutes, the path was a sea of red mud, and as I passed through the dense tree area, I was attacked by an assailant."

"What! You mean someone physically attacked you?" asked Karl anxiously.

"Yes. A man attacked me from behind and wrestled me to the ground. He tried to strangle me!" Sharon felt a lump in her throat as she attempted to go on. Her mouth was dry and she felt her heart beating forcefully.

"Oh my God! Are you alright, Sharon? Were you injured?"

"The storm was my salvation, because as I fell with him, both of us were soaked with mud and his grip on my throat became loose. I was able to fend him off with my umbrella and run for help."

"Who was it?"

"I don't know. He was wearing some type of a mask and he was never caught. I have related this story to local law enforcement here as well, and they will be watching over me for a while."

"I don't know what to say, Sharon."

"I'll be alright Dad, don't worry."

"Do you want me to come down and stay with you for a while?" "No, Dad, that won't be necessary, but thanks anyhow." Sharon was attempting to appear brave, but inside she was shaking. They talked for a while and she told him all about the Olympic events she had seen. After a while, Karl brought his daughter up to date with his life and what he was doing professionally.

"Sharon, last week the big news was about the hepatitis that was endemic to Europe and now has spread to South America and Africa. It seems that a new strain of the virus has developed through a mutation and it has a predilection for children. Evidently adults seem to have some immunity to this particular strain, but kids are rapidly succumbing to it."

"Are they dying in the acute phase of the illness?"

"No, they seem to go into the chronic form of the disease and develop cirrhosis."

"So the only chance for survival is a liver transplant."

"Right, but you know the problem there better than anyone."

"Unfortunately, I do. Not enough donors!"

"By the way, the paper also said that World Health Care, the HMO, was investing millions of dollars in an unnamed drug company who was attempting to develop a vaccine. The epidemiologists say this new strain of virus will eventually spread worldwide. Because of the twenty percent fatality rate, they anticipate that immunization will become mandatory throughout the world."

"That's interesting—we get a lot of World Health's transplant patients."

"Well Sharon, call me in a few days so I can be sure you're okay."

"Fine Dad, I will. Don't worry." She hung up the phone and walked to the TV, where she turned on the news.

▲ ▲ ▲

Kevin Knight had been a private investigator for fifteen years, and operated out of his office in Los Angeles. In the past, he had worked for James Foxworthy and always "got his man." On one occasion, he had been hired to seek out information on a doctor who was on staff at TWMC and was suspected of both personal drug abuse as well as issuing prescriptions for controlled substances to patients without proper indications. Kevin had been able to gather substantial evidence against the doctor, and when presented with it, the doctor left town. Foxworthy was delighted to avoid the negative publicity of that doctor practicing within the halls of TWMC, because many potential benefactors of TWMC might have been lost had the story been published in any form. Foxworthy showed his gratitude by including a five-thousand-dollar bonus in the final payment to Kevin. Kevin never forgot it, and whenever Foxworthy needed a favor, he was only too eager to please. He wrote notes on his pad as Foxworthy rapidly summarized what was needed. He was given all the available information at hand and promised to begin immediately. A moment later, Doctor Dell's personnel file came over the fax. Kevin sat at his desk and began to read the file. Over the next few days, he called and visited many people to inquire about Dell. All he could find was that she was well thought of, and her peers had nothing but the highest praise and admiration for her talents. Everyone commented about her extreme compassion for children.

This latter fact was confirmed when he personally interviewed the Director of Medical Education at the hospital where she had done her internship. Although this type of information was kept under lock and key, Kevin had used his phony ID, which identified him as an FBI agent. He convinced the director that he was performing a background check for security clearance. He said Sharon was being considered for a position with the government. She was joining a research team that was located within the CDC in Atlanta, and the nature of the work was classified. He was a pro at conning people and he had confidence that it would work because it had always been successful in the past.

Kevin was right as usual and gathered a great deal of data about Doctor Dell. By the seventh day, he had compiled a dossier and personally typed it on his PC. On that day, he hand delivered it to James Foxworthy's office and was rewarded with a check for six thousand dollars. The extra thousand took care of his expenses for the week very nicely.

~ *10* ~

BARRY'S STORY

F oxworthy perused the report and called Mike Rome to alert him that it was ready. Mike asked for the report to be delivered by special messenger to Doctor Paul Cook at the Research Center and then called Cook to alert him that it was on the way.

Doctor Cook notified his colleague, Doctor Matson, as soon as the report was delivered, and they met in the research library to discuss the matter. Cook made a copy of the twelve-page dossier and gave it to Matson. Both sat and read the report carefully, and after ten minutes, they began their discussion.

Victor was first to speak. "Paul, I think there may be something here we can hang our hat on," he said with confidence in his voice.

"Are you referring to her common characteristic that everyone comments upon?"

"If you mean Sharon's dedication and compassion to children, I am," answered Paul in a tone of voice that indicated he was peeved that Matson had seen the potential flaw also. Paul had an extremely strong ego, which he sought to protect at all costs. This jealousy led to the game of one-upmanship that they both participated in to see who would come up with a solution first. The game was repeated in everything they did. He believed in a saying he once observed on a T-shirt, *Second place is the first loser.*

"Her strong dedication and fervor about kids may be something we can use to our advantage."

"If we should allow her to actually see with her own eyes what we have on the third floor here, she may quiet down and understand that the lives of children are at stake," said Paul.

Victor stroked his chin and sat back in his chair. "You know, perhaps this was meant to happen now. The spread of the atypical hepatitis virus from Europe to other continents and the strong potential for it to spread to the U.S.A. might be just enough for her to go about her work and forget her crusade."

"She won't have anything to crusade about if we confide in her," said Paul, looking askance.

"Do I hear you suggesting that we tell her *everything* we are doing here?" asked Victor.

"Well, why not, if we are going to let her observe the fruits of our genetic research?" answered Paul. "Once she knows that part of our research, she might as well know it all."

"I guess so. If she blows the whistle on us, it will all come out anyhow," said Victor.

"We have got to make her see that the good far outweighs any of the negatives, which are really only two," said Paul with conviction.

"We are testing drugs without FDA approval, and we are actively involved in genetic engineering without big brother's sanction," said Victor quietly.

"When you put it like that, Victor, it doesn't appear to be that bad, especially when we can show the lives that we have saved with our products," said Paul, nodding at his colleague as if to ask for his approval.

"Well, I guess you ought to report our suggestion to Mike Rome, and if he goes for it, he'll send it on to the TWMC board."

"Yes, I'll do that right away. We will probably be hearing from them soon."

Mike relayed the suggestion that Doctor Dell be allowed to visit the research facilities with the notion that she would be amply impressed and her compassion would be great enough so as to induce her to forget about Linda Korn's case.

The board of directors was contacted individually about the proposal to allow Sharon to meet with the research department and tour the facility. They were unanimous in their decision to approve the plan. Barry Swenz was elected to approach Sharon with the idea but was cautioned not to say more than necessary to get her to consent to visit the research center. Needless to say, Barry wasn't very happy about being delegated the task, but he had no alternative. He called Sharon's secretary and arranged an appointment in her office the next day at 2 p.m. Barry was very anxious about the meeting. He knew he couldn't take the chance of disclosing information that might be damaging, yet he had to pique Sharon's interest enough to make her want to make the visit. That night, he didn't rest well.

At two o'clock sharp, Barry walked into Sharon's office. "Hello Sharon, good to see you again. How is everything going?"

"Fine, Barry, what brings you here?" she asked coyly.

"Let me guess. You found the operative reports on Linda!" She stared directly into his eyes until he turned away. After an eternity, he raised his eyes to hers and spoke. "Sharon, I want to talk to you about that situation as well as other aspects which have a direct relation to Linda Korn."

"Fine, I'm all ears!" she answered in earnest.

"A few years ago, I was asked to participate in a joint venture clinical research project that involved two large medically related companies. The research involved the development of an anti-rejection drug that seemed to have promise. It had been tested on research animals but not on man at that time, and the FDA placed a hold on all applications for reasons known only to them. The company was certain the drug would be a success; however, clinical testing was the next stage and they did not have the approval to do so. At that time, if you recall, the available anti-rejection drugs were often unsuccessful. As a result, many patients either died or underwent a second organ transplant because of rejection."

"Tell me Barry, which drug company did the research?"

Barry weighed his response before answering. On one hand, if he disclosed the name of the company, Sharon would be armed with potentially damaging information should she decide to walk away from the visit. But on the other, Bently's reputation was such that it was the industry's acknowledged leader in anti-rejection drug research. It had been responsible for saving the lives of thousands of people all over the world, and Sharon would be well aware of this. He quickly decided he would tell her. "Bently Drug Company," he answered.

Sharon's mouth literally dropped and her eyes widened. "You mean to tell me that Bently asked you to administer a drug not yet approved?" she said in disbelief.

"I'm afraid that is the truth," Barry replied, pursing his lips while shaking his head in anguish. "But it was done to save lives," he quickly amended, hoping to gain some sympathy from Sharon. Sharon rubbed her eyes with her hands and sighed. Barry was quick to catch the signal of compassion from the woman's body language. He knew he had to hit her with the hard facts if he was to gain her sympathy totally.

"I want to give you some facts regarding transplantation of organs in the United States, some of which you may already know. Please bear with me. In 1988, there were 12,786 transplants performed, and in 1989, there were 13,471. In 1990, '91, and '92, about 16,000 transplants were performed per year, and there was an increase of 1,000 per year after that. These were divided among the organs like this. About fifty percent were kidney, twenty percent liver, ten percent heart, and the rest were pancreas, lung, bowel, and heart-lung transplants. As of this year, the U.S. waiting list statistics include almost 50,000 registered patients waiting for an organ transplant. In 1995, almost 4,000 patients died while awaiting an organ transplant. Prior to 1995, the death rate while awaiting an organ transplant was 1,700 patients a year."

"Yes, I am well aware of these statistics Barry, but there is an additional fact which explains the doubling of those dying last year. Many transplant centers placed their transplants on hold because so many were having rejections; therefore, it took that much longer for a patient to get their organ. The longer an end-stage organ patient has to wait, the more likelihood there will be complications."

"Absolutely, and that leads me to the next point. Bently convinced me of the need to act swiftly to obtain results of clinical trials with their new drug they call KZ67. They showed me documents from all the medical centers and governments in Europe. These, without exception, said they would be willing to allow clinical testing in their countries, but Bently wanted to have it all done here because they were already set up for it in the U.S. In addition, they knew once the drug was accepted in Europe as a result of the U.S. research, the politicians here could be coerced into getting the FDA to quickly accept the drug. When that happened, they were going to change all the dates of the studies so they would be able to present large numbers of American patients that were treated with KZ67 in a shorter period of time, thereby complying with the FDA's regulation regarding the vast number of patients required for such a clinical trial."

"My God, you were helping them determine the clinical efficacy of KZ67 within this hospital! How was that possible? You had to keep records, and most of the patients were HMO insured. Weren't they suspicious? I know they do chart audits and closely review their hospitalized patients. How could your clinical trials escape our hospital's Pharmacy and Therapeutics Committee scrutiny?"

Barry swallowed hard. His mouth was dry. *I never expected*

her to tie in the HMO and the hospital. How am I going to explain this without having to tell her everything? Barry knew he was digging the pit bigger with each attempt to cover up the truth by errors of omission. She stared at him with a look of exasperation, and he knew he was losing her. He had to come clean and appeal to her altruistic feelings. Then, and only then, would he stand a chance of convincing her to at least visit the research center. After that, it would be up to Cook and Matson.

"Sharon, what I am about to divulge to you is extremely confidential. I want your word that you will not reveal any of it to a soul." Sharon thought for a brief moment. She knew this was her only chance to get to the bottom of the mystery that had plagued her both mentally and physically. She thought of the attack she had sustained while in Atlanta and shuddered. "You have my word," she said solemnly. Barry breathed a deep sigh of relief. "As you are aware, a few years ago there was an epidemic of hepatitis confined to Europe. The virus then underwent a mutation and spread throughout the rest of the world. It had a predilection for children, and the mortality rate was high. World Health Care HMO, who insures worldwide, was getting hit hard financially with the costs of caring for these patients. They formed an alliance with Genome Corporation to expedite the research in hopes of producing an antigen that could be used worldwide to immunize against the hepatitis virus and even possibly the discovery of an agent that would kill the virus as well. The other aspect of research was to intensify the clinical research on KZ67 in hopes that they could sell it to Europe and then the U.S. Their problem was that there was no place to do the clinical research on this anti-rejection drug. They needed controlled studies over a two-year period of time. These companies came to TWMC and offered a lot of money if the board of directors would allow the research to be carried out here."

Sharon's eyes grew wide as she fathomed the meaning of all she heard. Barry continued, "I was asked to do the clinic research on the KZ67. I followed the patients and gave them their drugs. I measured the parameters of liver, kidney, and hemopoietic function for two years after their transplants."

"That explains why all the postoperative transplants were assigned to you. I imagine you kept secret records on each patient then."

"Yes, I had to submit them to the research team per their protocol."

"Were there any patients who met with untoward results?"

"None. All the patients had excellent outcomes. There were no measurable side effects of KZ67, and at the end of two years, all patients were taken off the drug. They were followed for a time thereafter and everything appeared normal."

"There was not one single case of rejection during the drug treatment or after?"

"That's right. This is a miracle drug that neutralizes the body's immune system with specific reference to its ability to cause organ rejection."

"Do you mean to tell me these transplant patients are off all immunosuppressive drugs after a few years?" asked Sharon with amazement. She knew the statistics for organ rejection were high. At the end of three years, there was a 25 percent rejection rate for kidney transplants and 40 percent for liver transplants. If the patients were fortunate, a second transplant was performed. KZ67 offered life without the possibility of another surgery or death from complications of a rejection causing organ failure.

"God, that's great!" she said with fervor.

"They are not only taken off KZ67, but are eventually taken off steroids as well!" responded Barry with obvious pride. "As a result of this research, KZ67 is now being marketed in Europe as well as the rest of the world. Just recently, the application for FDA approval to perform clinical research in the United States was submitted."

"That's perjury. You plan to include all the patients you have already studied for more than two years by changing the dates so it would appear they are being studied now."

"Yes. In that manner, we will be able to document the required number of patients over the ensuing two years. If we had to start from scratch, it would take us five years to get enough patient data."

"So what. Why not do it legally?"

"Because the sale of this drug is important to the companies. They are depending upon the sales to support a large part of the other research currently going on." He paused as he realized he might have just opened another can of worms, but it was too late.

"What other research are they doing?

"I am not privy to that information, Sharon." Sharon was amazed and angry at the same time. Amazed that KZ67 was truly a miracle drug, if it did indeed alter the immune system in such a manner that organ rejection could be overcome in only two years and there was no detrimental effect on the rest of the body's immune system. But angry over the planned subterfuge directed against the FDA. She was well aware of the short-comings of the federal red tape agency, but they did serve as a safeguard for the public, despite moving at a snail's pace. "Tell me Barry, how is the research coming on a hepatitis antigen?"

"From what I hear, they are very close. One of the most important tools they had was the actual livers." Barry had to be careful now, and he knew it. "The company had a re-search lab in Europe that received the diseased livers from those dying of the disease. They were also fortunate in that the European governments were supportive of their research efforts. They had always approved drugs with less red tape than the FDA required. It stemmed from their basic belief in the common good produced by medical research. Over the years, they had acquired vast experience by the use of drug approval at early stages of clinical research. It was a rare occurrence when a drug had to be taken off the market be-cause of undesirable side effects. These governments gave their blessing to companies involved in producing medicines to help the people of the world.

"Having a continuous supply of hepatitis-infected livers was instrumental to diminishing the time required to study and isolate the virus. They've come up with new techniques and been very successful in that regard."

Sharon sat quietly and mulled over the facts she had just heard. There was something missing or out of place. She thought a moment longer, and then it hit her. "What has all this got to do with Linda Korn?"

"I am not at liberty to discuss that with you, but I have been asked by the Research Lab partners if you would meet them at their facility so they might explain it all to you in detail."

"They want me to meet with them? I don't know much about research. Why would they want to speak with me about it?"

"Evidently, there are many aspects to the research program they want you to know about."

Her inquisitive nature got the better part of her. "Who are the main researchers?"

"Doctor Victor Matson is the Chief of Bently Drug's Research Program, and Paul Cook is the Chief of Genome's research section. They are both directing the research program."

Sharon gasped. She knew these men's reputation. They were at the top of the elite ladder in medical research. What was more, she had read many of their published articles over the years and respected them greatly for their knowledge and dedication. Now she was presented with an opportunity to meet them face to face. How could she possibly refuse? "Alright, I will meet with them. When will we do it?

"You set the date and time, and I will confirm it with them."

"Next Monday morning will be fine."

Barry stood up and approached her desk. "I will get back to you tomorrow with a confirmation on the meeting. Thanks Sharon." He walked out of her office feeling uplifted, leaving Sharon wondering why he had thanked her.

The next day, Sharon received word from Barry that the meeting was on for Monday morning. He told her that he would meet her in the TWMC parking lot at 7 a.m. and drive her to the research facilities himself.

-11-

THE FIRST CLUE

Karl Dell was sent by the DOC to do a field audit at Squire Hospital in San Diego. The state's computer data had identified an extreme departure from normal with regard to the number of hospital admissions for repeated transplant surgeries on HMO patients.

Entering the spacious hospital atrium, Karl was directed to the medical records department. The medical record department staff had already been asked to collect certain data, as well as to pull the patients' charts for audit.

After identifying himself to the medical record librarian, he was led to a small room where all the charts were neatly piled. Reams of computer data were also lying next to the charts.

"Thank you. I'll call you if I have any questions," said Karl in a friendly manner. The medical record librarian took her leave and closed the door behind her. Karl began to audit each chart individually. He placed clips on the pages he wanted copied and made numerous notes on a legal pad.

It wasn't very long before he realized that most of the

patients were admitted from other parts of California and a large number were from other states also. There was no law that would preclude patients from another state or another part of California from coming to Squire, but it was sure strange. These were all managed care patients who were insured by World Health Care HMO, and he knew that often an HMO would contract with one large hospital center for its more esoteric therapy and procedures. *Perhaps that is the reason,* thought Karl.

He dug deeper into each chart to see if there was any other common thread. He noticed that the number of patients who underwent second transplants was twice the national average. What bothered him the most was there were a number of patients who had initially had a kidney transplant, then three to four years later they'd required a liver transplant. All the patients that had the second transplant surgery were not on any immunological suppressant drug therapy. He knew enough about transplant surgery to know that the body would reject a transplanted organ too many times even when the patient *was* on an immunosuppressant drug regimen, let alone not on any at all. He thought he was missing something, so he again reviewed some forty charts to see if he could find a clue. He was unsuccessful in doing so. The medical records also seemed to be incomplete in terms of the postoperative care of the patients. While the records revealed that steroids had been administered, no other immunosuppressant was recorded. Yet all the charts stated that immunosuppressant therapy was given according to the HMO protocol. *I need to ask Sharon about this. She might have an answer.* He gathered his belongings and thanked the medical record librarian again and started to leave the hospital. Then he stopped abruptly and turned around, facing the librarian. "Would all medical records accompanying patients from either a hospital transfer or from their primary care doctor be placed in the medical charts?"

"Yes, they would," she answered.

Well, that ends that, he thought. *I thought perhaps the transfer medical data might have been filed separately and would explain why the patients weren't taking immunosuppressant drug therapy.*

–12–

CLONES IN THE GARDEN

Sharon was in her parked car at 7 a.m. on Monday morning awaiting Barry Swenz. He arrived promptly, leaned over from the driver's seat, and opened the passenger door for her. She entered and put on her seat belt.

"I smell coffee," she said, looking at Barry.

"You sure do—it's in the bag at your feet with all the fixings." She opened the white bag and removed the styrofoam cup, pleased to see it was a large one. She recalled how she hated small styrofoam cups, but a large one she could tolerate. Next to the coffee was a wrapped cinnamon roll. "Is this for me?" Sharon asked.

"It's all yours," he replied with a grin.

"That was very thoughtful of you. I love cinnamon rolls."

"I know you do," Barry said spontaneously without realizing it.

Sharon looked at him with her head slightly cocked to the side and asked, "And how would you know that?"

Barry began to panic. He knew everything about her from the private investigator's dossier he had read, but he couldn't let her know that. *What an idiot I am. I talk too much.*

"I meant to say I guessed you would," he answered in a very self-assured and positive manner. Placing the car in drive, he pulled out of the parking lot. In a few minutes, he was on the San Bernardino Freeway headed west to Los Angeles.

Sharon sipped her coffee and munched on the cinnamon role with gusto. It had been at least two months since she'd had one. *Too many calories,* she thought, *but what the heck, today I feel adventurous!*

"Looks like you're sure enjoying that roll!"

"You bet I am. I was famished this morning, and since I got up late, I didn't get a chance to eat. Where are we going, Barry?"

"The research center is located in Malibu. I have only been there twice, but I remember the way."

"Good, because I'm sure I would get lost in that area." They drove with the radio tuned to KFI, where the morning talk show host was screaming at someone foolhardy enough to call in with an answer to the host's previously posed question. The only problem was that the answer was not acceptable to the host. He was known for his screaming antics that for some unknown reason attracted many listeners to the station.

Barry was the first to comment. "This guy gets my blood boiling sometimes with his gimmicks."

"What do you mean by gimmicks?" asked Sharon naively.

"Well, let me give you an example," he answered as he

reached forward to turn the volume down. "Remember when Ronald Reagan announced he had Alzheimer's?"

"Yes, about a year ago, I think."

"That's right. One of the station's comics wrote a song about him, and it had lyrics that were appalling. They said Reagan was talking to trees and other very demeaning things about his behavior. They managed to incorporate lyrics describing all the severe memory deficits seen with Alzheimer's. I really took offense with it, and I'm still angered."

"I agree with you. To make fun of someone who is suffering from an illness is horrible, but it is twice as bad when you do it to a former president of the United States." "That's my feeling, exactly."

"Then why do you listen to the jerk?"

"I don't know, I guess I like the feeling of control I get when I can shut him off."

"Whatever turns you on, Barry!"

"A few years ago, there was another loudmouth on the same station who sounded to me like he was a manic. He was eventually fired, and I was delighted. Now that I think about it, I used to listen to him also and bitch all the while. I remember the pleasure I derived whenever I shut the radio off. I hear him on another station occasionally now and laugh. It's interesting that since his change in stations, his entire demeanor has changed. The manic aggressive behavior isn't there anymore. I'd bet anything he was treated for manic depression."

"Sounds like you're a talk show enthusiast."

"Whenever I'm in the car, I listen to news or talk shows.

If it gets out of control, I shut it off and it doesn't bother me." They were now on Kanaan Road headed west to Malibu. In a few miles, Barry turned to the right and followed a street to the end where it ran into an unpaved road. As they drove on, large signs appeared advising them that they were on private property and were trespassing unless they had business with the research facility.

In short order, they approached the kiosk. The area was enclosed by a twelve-foot-high fence with razor wire at the top. Large towers could be seen at intervals along the fence line.

"What is your business?" asked the guard.

"Doctors Dell and Swenz to see Doctors Cook and Matson."

"May I see some ID, please." At the request, both occupants withdrew their driver's licenses and handed them to the guard, who took them and walked back into the kiosk. He spoke on the phone and returned to the vehicle, handing the licenses to Barry. "Thank you. Please park your car in the inside lot to the right, and a guard will escort you to your meeting."

Sharon raised her eyes in wonder as she looked at Barry. He drove through the gates and parked in the lot as instructed. A utility vehicle pulled up in back of them and waited.

"I can't believe all the security here," said Sharon. "They actually escort you to the building?" She pointed her finger at the research center.

"That's the way they do it here. Let's go." They exited the car and got into the waiting utility vehicle. The vehicle drove off toward the building about a quarter mile away. They were escorted inside, where they each received a visitor's pass, but only after they'd each had their photo taken.

"Just like the DMV," said Sharon. The DMV took photos that were instantaneously available but not always complimentary. The clerk attached the photos to the badges, and then the guard led them to the elevator, which quickly deposited them on the second floor. They were led into a large conference room where the two researchers were seated. Dr. Cook was wearing a long white coat and stood six feet tall. He was a handsome, clean-shaven man in his late fifty's with a full head of brown hair graying at the temples. His aura exuded a friendly demeanor, and he was the first to greet Sharon. "I am very happy to meet you, Dr. Dell. I have heard the finest of reports about you." He took both her hands in his and squeezed gently. "I want you to meet my colleague, Dr. Matson."

"Dr. Dell, your reputation precedes you. I am happy to meet you." Matson extended his hand to Sharon. The doctor was of average height, with pattern baldness and a medium build. He wore a neatly trimmed beard and mustache, which were modestly gray. His eyes were brown and they seemed to twinkle. He was also wearing the apparel of the senior researcher, the status symbol of the long white coat. Sharon smiled as she thought of her past training. She had always been told the length of the white coat in medicine was directly proportional to seniority. Interns and residents always wore short white jackets, signifying their low position on the totem pole.

"The feeling is mutual, Dr. Matson. I have read some of your papers and Dr. Cook's in the medical literature. I admire you both immensely!"

"Thank you for those kind words, Dr. Dell," said Matson, obviously pleased with the accolade.

"Please sit down, Doctor, May we offer you some coffee?" asked Cook.

"I will take a cup of coffee with one Equal if you don't mind."

"And what about you, Dr. Swenz?" Cook asked.

"Coffee, black will be fine." Cook poured the coffee from a silver pot into two large mugs. He handed one to Barry, and after adding the sweetener, he handed the other to Sharon. She sat down and sipped her coffee. The room was large enough to easily contain a long table that seated at least twelve. At the front of the room was a large chalkboard that had recently been washed. It was streaked, but the black color glistened. Barry sat next to her and Cook and Matson took the seats directly across from them. They had discussed the seating arrangements between themselves earlier and decided it would be best for them to sit directly across from Sharon. If they sat at the head of the table, it might have created the illusion of control.

"Dr. Dell, we have asked you here to get your thoughts on a few items, and we hope to explain our research program to you," said Matson.

"I am delighted to be here. I have a few questions of my own."

"Dr. Dell, I am going to assume you have little knowledge

in the field of recombinant genetics, and I will attempt, with Dr. Cook's aid, to outline our program."

"You have made a correct assumption, Dr. Matson. The only genetics I recall is the simple Mendelian genetics."

Dr. Cook smiled in approval of her admission to his suspicion.

"Let me start with some definitions," said Matson. "Genes are segments of DNA that code for specific proteins. Another way of looking at it is that the code is a plan, which instructs the cell as to how to make a certain protein. A gene is made of a segment of DNA that contains exons that are separated by introns. The intron is a noncoding segment, while the exon is the segment of the gene responsible for coding for the production of specific proteins. The exon is that template part of a gene that yields a messenger ribonucleic acid (mRNA) product that codes for a specific protein. mRNA differs from DNA in that it is single-stranded, contains ribose as the sugar, and substitutes uracil, one of the base pairs, for thymine. An intron is the part of the gene not represented in mature mRNA, and therefore, noncoding for protein. The codon is a sequence of three base pairs in RNA or DNA that codes for a specific amino acid. The genes are located on chromosomes, and the entire genetic complement is called a genome. The chromosome consists of protein and DNA. There are twenty-three pairs of chromosomes in man, and each chromosome contains many genes. Molecular biology's dogma is that information flows from DNA to RNA to protein. RNA is assembled with the aid of the DNA template and is responsible for making protein molecules. "Each molecule of DNA has a deoxyribose sugar backbone, and each deoxyribose is attached to one of four nucleic acids, which we call nuclear bases. The DNA consists of two deoxyribose strands in a double alpha helix with the nucleic acids on the inside and the nuclear bases paired by hydrogen bonding of adenine with thymine and cytosine with guanine. A base pair is either adenine-guanine or cytosine-thymine, the nucleic acid of one chain paired with the facing nucleic acid of the other chain. This is called complimentary base pairing. Visualize a ladder. If you were to hold it at one end and turn the opposite end, it would be twisted like a corkscrew. The rungs of the ladder are the base pairs, while the sides are the sugar and phosphate molecules. A fragment of DNA is measured by the numbers of base pairs. It is estimated that humans have three billion base pairs. The nucleotide is the basic building block of DNA. It is composed of the sugar, the deoxyribose, a phosphate group, and a nucleic acid base. Have I lost you yet?" asked Matson.

"I have been taking notes, and I think I follow you," replied Sharon.

"Fine then. I will ask Dr. Cook to pick up the discussion in just a moment. As I told you, there are three billion base pairs or six billion nucleotides in each human genome. The human has somewhere between 100,000 and 300,000 genes, and the entire genetic language is written in only four letters: A, C, G, and T in DNA, and A, C, G, and U in RNA. All the nucleotides are abbreviated using the first letter of their name. G for Guanine, A for Adenine, T for Thymine, C for Cytosine, and U for Uracil. These are the nucleotides that make up the base pairs. The language contains only three-letter words or codons. The genome is divided into twenty-three pairs of chromosomes contained in each cell. The gametes or egg and sperm contain half this number. There are only sixty-four combinations that can result from four nucleotides and three-letter words. I realize this is an awful lot of information to digest, but it is essential you have an overview to help you understand the research we do here." He paused and asked Cook to continue.

"I shall begin with the cloning procedure. A clone is a genetically identical cell or organism derived from a single ancestor by asexual or parasexual methods. What I am about to describe is the way in which cloning is accomplished in research universally. A circular segment of DNA, called a plasmid, is obtained from a bacterium into which the DNA to be cloned will be spliced. The next step is the use of restriction enzymes to cleave both the plasmid and the appropriate segment of genomic DNA. This leaves the fragment DNA in sort of a letter *c* configuration. This is followed by the use of another enzyme, DNA ligase, which splices the DNA section of interest with the exposed ends of the plasmid that closes the circle. The result is a *recombinant* DNA molecule. The word recombinant then refers to the recombination of DNA segments one wishes to clone and the bacterial plasmid. The recombinant molecules are then introduced back into the bacterial cells, where the bacteria containing the recombinant DNA multiply. If the DNA spliced into the plasmid was a gene, the bacteria begin producing the protein coded for by that gene. This technology has many clinical applications today. This is the way in which insulin is now produced. The bacteria continue to code for the insulin protein because they are told to do so by the DNA in the gene that was originally of human origin.

"What are restriction enzymes, and where do they come from?" asked Sharon. "Good question, Dr. Dell. I can see you have been following this," answered Cook, trying to be complimentary to her. "A restriction enzyme is a protein that is able to identify certain sequences of nucleotide code letters and to cut the DNA strand wherever it finds them. For example, the restriction enzyme Eco RI will cut DNA whenever it confronts the sequence GAATTC. It always cuts the DNA strand between the G and A.

"At least one hundred restriction enzymes have been identified in bacteria. Each enzyme cuts a different DNA sequence, and their purpose is to defend bacteria from viruses by recognizing sequences of nucleotides. One enzyme recognizes GAATC within an invading virus and severs the DNA. Because of this, the virus can't replicate, so they die without killing the host bacteria. The bacteria lacks this DNA sequence, so the enzyme can't do any damage to itself. The human genetic complement contains every restriction enzyme sequence known to man; therefore, we don't have restriction enzymes. If we had them, our own DNA would be cut in the attempt to kill invading viruses.

"Now that we are armed with the tool of recombinant DNA technology, researchers are able to clone specific segments of DNA and identify the sequence of base pairs in those segments. As such, the search for the location of the gene went into high gear. We have been able to identify the location of genes by analyzing the type of protein coded for by the gene present in the DNA. Modern medicine has been able to identify the location of the genes that cause sickle cell anemia, Tay Sachs disease, hypercholesterolemia and hemophilia. All of these genetic illnesses are the result of abnormal proteins. There are more than three thousand known genetic diseases that defy location today.

"Research advanced when a method to identify a marker on a segment of DNA to approximate the location of a gene was discovered. As the search continued, with the use of restriction enzymes to cut DNA fragments, an interesting curiosity was observed. When analogous segments of DNA were taken from different individuals, and cut by the same restriction enzyme, the resulting DNA fragments were of different lengths. This suggested that there had to be slight differences between human nucleotide sequences. It has been shown that about one in five hundred base pairs are different between individuals. The molecular biologists claim that, at the DNA level, all of us are ninety-nine percent identical. This difference in the lengths of similar DNA sections has been named *restriction fragment length polymorphisms*, or RFLPs. Geneticists call them *reflips*. It was also discovered that these RFLPs were genetically transmitted through generations. The use of reflips became the dominant instrument in the search for the location of genes. RFLPs are used as markers on chromosomes when trying to map the location of a gene and are useful in determining inheritance patterns of disease. I think, at this point, I'll ask Dr. Matson to talk about the polymerase chain reaction."

"I'm amazed at all I've heard to this point," said Sharon enthusiastically. "What about you, Barry?

"To be brutally honest, this is way over my head. I follow some of it, but I'd need some study time to really understand all of it."

"Your difficulty is appreciated," answered Cook, and he gestured to Matson that the floor was his.

"The reaction is called PCR, and it was devised about ten years ago. Cloning to detect specific DNA sequences is very time consuming. The PCR allows us to produce enormous numbers of copies of a specific DNA sequence without resorting to cloning. DNA polymerasecan be directed to synthesize a specific region of DNA, as well as amplify it by the use of primers, which direct the starting points for the DNA synthesis. DNA polymerase is an enzyme that brings single nucleotides into a DNA molecule. PCR amplification is used to detect mutations, monitor cancer therapy, and detect bacterial and viral infections by isolating the DNA segments of interest from minute quantities and reproducing them exponentially. The aim is to detect the rare cancer or infected cell so as to guide further therapy. PCR techniques are capable of detecting as few as one cancer cell in ten million normal cells. To detect the AIDS virus, HIV, PCR primers are made for RNA sequences in the virus, and a PCR is carried out with DNA extracted from blood cells.

"Now, I want to discuss RNA. DNA cannot act as the template for protein, because almost all the DNA is restricted within the nucleus of the cell; however, all the protein synthesis occurs in the cytoplasm of the cell. It follows then that a gene encoded on the DNA must be transferred to the cytoplasm of the cell. The molecule that carries this message is messenger RNA (mRNA). When mRNA is assembled, uracil always base pairs with the adenine of the DNA template.

"Transcription is the synthesis of single-stranded messenger RNA from a gene. In the initiation of transcription, the two chains of the double helix come apart with one of the strands copied into its RNA complement, which then travels from the chromosome to the cytoplasm where it sequences the assembly of amino acids into proteins. In transcription, exact complementary bases are made from mRNA that are determined by the DNA template. The A, T, C, and G of DNA pair with the U, A, G, and C in mRNA respectively. Prior to mRNA exiting the cell nucleus, the introns are spliced out. Introns are non-coding and therefore don't contribute to making protein molecules in the cytoplasm. In the cytoplasm, mRNA translates the nucleotide language of nucleic acids into the amino acid language of proteins. This is known as translation.

The RNA molecules serve as templates that order the assembly of amino acids into the polypeptide chains. You do recall that all proteins are made from amino acids, don't you?"

Matson smiled congenially and went on with his soliloquy. "Always remember, molecular biology's dogma is that information flows from DNA to RNA to protein. We now return to what I told you earlier when I first spoke to you about codons. The groups of nucleotides that code for an amino acid are called codons. They are a sequence of three base pairs in RNA or DNA and are also called the triplet codon. For example, the codon UUU codes for the production of the amino acid phenylalanine, UCU specifies serine, UAU specifies tyrosine and the codon UGU specifies cysteine."

Matson handed out a printed paper showing the genetic code that he had just discussed. Sharon took the text eagerly while Barry didn't show the same interest. He placed it on the desk without looking at it at all. He was somewhat buried with the volume of data. Sharon looked at the document before her and was intrigued. "May we have a moment to read this please?" she asked.

"Why, of course you may," replied Matson. He sat down at the table and poured a cup of coffee. "This is hard stuff to get all in a short time," he said as he sipped the coffee.

"Could you explain this chart further?"

"Certainly. First let me explain about the position of the bases in a codon. Remember that a nucleotide is comprised of deoxyribose, the sugar, a phosphate, and a nucleic acid base. Every nucleic acid chain has a direction defined by the position of its sugar-phosphate backbone. The phosphorous is linked to the 5 carbon of one sugar and the 3 carbon of the next sugar in the chain. Therefore one end is termed the 5' {5 prime} end and the other the 3' end. DNA and its nuclear acid sequences are written from left to right, which is from the 5' to the 3' end. This is the direction of the transcription process, which I will speak to in a moment. The end of the chain that terminates with the 5 carbon atom is named the 5' end, and the end terminating with the 3 carbon atom is the 3' end. All RNA and DNA chains are assembled in the 5'-to-3' direction."

He projected an outline on the screen from his computer and gave Sharon a printed copy as well.

The Messenger RNA Genetic Code

First Position 5' end	Second Position				Third Position 3' end
	U	C	A	G	
	Phe	Ser	Tyr	Cys	U
	Phe	Ser	Tyr	Cys	C
U	Leu	Ser	Stop	Stop	A
	Leu	Ser	Stop	Trp	G
	Leu	Pro	His	Arg	U
C	Leu	Pro	His	Arg	C
	Leu	Pro	Gln	Arg	A
	Leu	Pro	Gln	Arg	G
	Ile	Thr	Asn	Ser	U
	Ile	Thr	Asn	Ser	C
A	Ile	Thr	Lys	Arg	A
	Met	Thr	Lys	Arg	G
	Val	Ala	Asp	Gly	U
	Val	Ala	Asp	Gly	C
G	Val	Ala	Glu	Gly	A
	Val	Ala	Glu	Gly	G

Amino Acid	Three-Letter Abbreviation	Amino Acid	Three-Letter Abbreviation
Serine	Ser	Tyrosine	Tyr
Cysteine	Cys	Tryptophane	Tr
Glycine	Gly	Proline	Pro
Histidine	His	Glutamine	Gln
Arginine	Arg	Isoleucine	Ile
Methionine	Met	Threonine	Thr
Asparagine	Asn	Lysine	Lys
Valine	Val	Alanine	Ala
Aspartic Acid	Asp	Glutamic Acid	Glu
Leucine	Leu		

~ 13 ~

INSIDE THE RNA MESSENGER AND DNA

"**N**ow if you will follow me on the Messenger RNA Genetic Code sheet I've given you, I will show you how to find the amino acid from the position of the bases in the codon. For example: the codon 5' AUG3' on messenger RNA specifies methionine, and CAU specifies histidine. You will notice that UAA, UAG, and UGA are termination signals. UUU specifies phenylalanine, UCU specifies serine, and UAU specifies tyrosine. Remember, all codons contain three successive nucleotides, which are a nucleic acid base, phosphate, and deoxyribose sugar. The nuclear bases again are AGTC, or in RNA, U is substituted for T. Many amino acids are specified by more than one codon, and as you can see, 61 of the possible 64 combinations of the three bases of a codon code for amino acids. The three combinations, UAA, UAG, and UGA, are stop codons. The signals for starting and stopping the synthesis of specific RNA molecules are encoded within DNA sequences.

"Any change in DNA sequence is one type of mutation. A change in a single nucleic acid base in a codon will result in the alteration of the protein, which will result in a loss or a change in function. Sickle Cell Anemia is the result of the substitution of a single base, {T} thymine for {A} adenine in the beta globulin gene.

"A proto-oncogene is a gene that has the potential to cause malignancy given the right set of circumstances. They encode proteins that participate in signal pathways, which relay the command to replicate. Some encode growth factors that are molecules that are themselves a signal to grow, while others encode growth factor receptors, and still others encode proteins that combine with growth factor receptors just inside the plasma membrane of the cell. I think I shall stop here."

Barry stared at Sharon and took a deep breath. "Are you ready for a quiz now?"

Sharon laughed aloud and was joined by Cook and Matson. "You have just acquired one semester of genetics in two hours, so don't feel badly."

"I am truly grateful for the enlightenment in this field. I never realized how much there was that I didn't ever know about genetics."

"Believe me, Dr. Dell," interrupted Cook, "that only scratched the surface. You can't believe the depth and breadth of this field. Every day, there is a new discovery that catapults all genetic research forward."

"Why don't we go to the lab and show you what we are doing in our research program," said Matson.

"Would you direct me to the nearest ladies room?"

"Certainly, just turn to the right outside this door," said Cook, pointing to the exit. "It's the first door on your right."

Sharon walked out of the room as the three doctors all rose from their seats.

"Well, what do you think Barry?" asked Matson.

"She sure is intrigued by all of it. I think it's a good sign."

"Well, we will find out in pretty short order, won't we?" replied Cook.

Sharon returned, and they all followed Cook and Matson out of the conference room. The entourage marched in twos to the end of a short hall, which was barricaded with a thick glass door. There was a large box implanted in the wall, and right above it was a slot for an ID card. Cook inserted the card and then placed his right hand over the glass on the box for a fingerprint identification match clearance. The door opened to reveal a guard stationed just inside, requesting that everyone sign a roster. He inspected the passes of the guests and then stepped aside. Sharon pulled Barry aside and asked him what was so important that required all the heavy-duty security. Barry was about to answer when Matson turned and addressed Sharon. "You are probably wondering about the extensive security precautions we have in place. Let me assure you, it is needed. We must protect the products of our research because, in this day and age, corporate stealing is very much alive and well. Many of our programs have taken years to get to their current stage, and if a scientific discovery were to be taken from us, we would suffer immense financial loss, not to mention the setback in research, some of which would take years to duplicate. Many of our competitors would love to know how we do things here. You see, we not only do the research, but we also have developed newer and quicker ways to perform various procedures. Dr. Matson and I have discovered methods that are superior to those used by our colleagues, and I might add we also are about ready to publish a new paper on oncogenes."

"I do understand your concerns, Dr. Cook," replied Sharon, nodding her head in agreement.

They entered a large room with many workers all in white jackets. The large area was divided into smaller spaces that housed research in bacteriology, biochemistry, immunology, oncology, and molecular genetics. Gas chromatographs, protein electrophoresis, gel electrophoresis, centrifuges, and massive computers were strategically placed throughout the lab, which encompassed at least five thousand square feet.

Matson and Cook led them through the busy area and stopped periodically to introduce an occasional employee. Cook mentioned that well over 90 percent of the employees had PhDs, while the rest had their Master's of Science degrees and were working toward their doctorates. The talent was immense, and both Barry and Sharon were duly impressed. After they completed the tour, they were led to the first floor, where the research animals were housed and cared for. Two veterinarians were in charge of that sector. They were shown hundreds of cages of mice, rats, and rabbits in one room. In another, they saw cats and dogs by the dozens, and still another room housed monkeys and chimpanzees. All the cages were spotless, with the grated floors open for drainage and cleansed hourly by an automatic system. In this manner, the catch floor of each animal's cage was continuously kept clean and therefore free from all odor. As if that weren't enough, the eight thousand square feet of cages were attended by eight animal assistants. At the rear of the caged area was a five-hundred-square-foot room, which housed all the latest surgical equipment.

Any hospital would have been proud to have such a modern operating room suite.

Sharon caught herself with her mouth wide open in astonishment. She imagined her awe and amazement to be akin to a person from South Dakota visiting New York City for the first time as they gaped awestruck at the skyscrapers.

"Okay folks, let's go to the elevators now and continue our excursion," said Matson as though he were a tour leader speaking to a group of children. They filed out of the lab and through the security-glass-gated door, then marched to the elevator. In a moment, the group was on the third floor. They were deposited into a large room, at the end of which was a giant, sealed door. Next to the door was another fingerprint scanner, and above the frame were three video cameras arranged in such a fashion that they were able to film the entire room. To the right of the door was mounted another camera at head level, and directly beneath it on the desk was a strange-looking device that analyzed and compared voice prints.

"The security system in place here is much more complex than the previous one, Dr. Dell," explained Dr. Cook.

"How so?" responded Sharon.

"Watch Dr. Matson as he enters the answers to the questions."

A computer was sitting next to the analyzer on the desk, and a menu was apparently walking Matson through the process of identification. After he entered his name and ID number, he was asked a number of questions about his personal life which required answering within twenty seconds. The computer randomly selected questions to ask from its database, which were acquired from each employee's personnel file. Questions were posed pertaining to family, interests, past employment, various important dates, names of relatives, and even on occasion a question asking the name of a specific past undergraduate or graduate course and the name of the professor who'd taught it. In this manner, it would be virtually impossible for someone to gain access who was not authorized to do so. As soon as the procedure was terminated, Cook went through the identical security clearance and then entered data into the computer on both guests. For non-employees, the pictures on their badges were scanned into the computer by a video scanner. Barry and Sharon were then asked to place their hands on the fingerprint scanner and answer three questions posed by the computer. Sharon was asked the names of her father and a previous chief of surgery, and the last four digits of her phone number, while similar questions were posed to Barry. At the conclusion, they were allowed to enter.

"Dr. Cook, how did the computer recognize Barry's and my fingerprints?" she inquired suspiciously.

"Very simply, Dr. Dell. While we were all downstairs, the coffee cups you and Dr. Swenz drank from supplied the prints. One of our people transferred the prints into the database, so by the time we arrived, the data was already loaded and could easily be compared with each of you."

Sharon was stunned. *What unmitigated gall.* She suddenly felt fearful.

They entered a darkened room that had three doors for exits, all of which were closed. Cook motioned them all through the first door and they found themselves standing in a room encompassing some four thousand square feet. Sharon was the first to speak. "What are those balloon-like things?"

She was staring at what appeared to be long rows of transparent balloons filled with fluid suspended from a superstructure. The fluid was semi-opaque, with lines of tubing exiting each balloon that connected to a long line of tubing running the length of each row. The rows were fifty feet long, and at the end of each row's tubing they joined another set of larger tubes that extended at right angles another thirty feet to a piece of machinery that broke the silence with its low-pitch murmur. Matson motioned to her to join him at the beginning of the first row. She responded quickly.

"I am going to turn on the lights now," he said, directing his remarks to Sharon, "and I will allow you both to walk through the room and make your observations. Afterward, Dr. Cook and I shall be delighted to answer your questions. I believe you will have no difficulty in finding questions to ask us." The room lightened with a flick of the switch. Sharon noticed that the fluid in the balloons was now translucent, and she walked to the first balloon and focused her vision on it. It took but a second, and she screamed, "Oh my God! It's a liver! I don't believe my own eyes. This is incredible!" She turned to Cook and Matson, who were standing at the wall of the room, watching her. Barry was standing in the second row, staring at the balloons.

"You are growing livers! How can you do that?" she asked excitedly.

Cook was first to answer. "Dr. Dell, we have developed a cloning method by which we can grow donor parts."

"But … how did you do this?"

"Please Dr. Dell, look at everything now and then we will explain it in more detail," pleaded Matson. "First, we will explain this operating system and then we will discuss the method by which we acquire the livers."

Sharon walked slowly along the row of balloons and saw that each had a liver suspended within that was surrounded by fluid. Each liver was also a different size, indicating various degrees of maturation. Numerous tubes were attached to the balloon base. Within most of these tubes was colorless fluid; however, in the smaller tubes, there was obvious blood being transported from the balloon along the maze of lines. Suddenly the thought hit her. *What was the blood doing, and how was it circulated?* She followed the tubes to the end of the row, where they connected to others that ran perpendicular to the three rows. Her eyes followed the red lines as they approached the equipment at the corner of the room. "Is that what I think it is?" asked Sharon.

"I'm sure it is. It is the latest heart-lung machine, the Pulmocor," replied Matson.

"It operates the same way here as in open heart surgery. The hepatic artery and vein are cannulated, and the vein drains the blood, which is propelled by the rollers you see at intervals all along the tubing. The venous line from each liver drains into one large venous line, which empties into a venous filter in a venous reservoir. Blood flows by gravity to a roller pump that squeezes the tube and propels the blood to the oxygenator. The oxygenator, or gas exchange module, is composed of hollow fibers specially created to assure a uniform blood flow around the fibers without stagnation. Oxygen is fed into the inlet port of the module along with Heparin to prevent coagulation and is then directed to flow inside these fibers, which are like long straws with much smaller openings. The carbon dioxide is removed, and the oxygen diffuses from the inside of these fibers to the surrounding blood bathing the fibers. The blood is then collected at the bottom of the reservoir and pumped with simple rollers back through the hepatic arteries, where it enters the liver and circulates throughout the organ, just as if it were pumped by a heart. You will notice that there is a highly efficient heat exchanger module that regulates the temperature of the fluid surrounding the blood tubing so that it is always at body temperature. It is foolproof and is even equipped with an alarm, which will sound should the volume of reservoir blood fall below a pre-designated level." He smiled at Sharon when he concluded.

"Dr. Matson, how can you pump the same blood through all the different livers?"

"Very good observation and question, Sharon. Dr. Cook and his crew discovered a method by which any blood can be used for this purpose. We used to use donated primate blood for this purpose, but since the life of the red blood cell is less than thirty days, and after that it doesn't carry oxygen that well, it must be replaced. We have also been able to produce red blood cells through genetic engineering. More about that later. I'm getting ahead of myself."

"The blood is safe then, and there won't be any hemolytic reactions?"

"Correct, because we clone type O Rh negative blood. Please look further at the other two rows." Sharon cast a questioning look at her mentor and nodded her head in agreement. She walked briskly to the middle row of balloon-like bags and gazed intently upon the first one. Like all the rest, it dangled from a superstructure, which resembled a giant light bulb with one noticeable difference. Many tubes were entering and exiting from the base like giant spaghetti and eventually joined larger ones as they meandered along to their final destination, where life-giving gasses were exchanged. Matson had explained that the reason for the fluid within the balloons that surrounded each organ was simply to handle the rest of the wastes of cellular metabolism. This bathing fluid was similar to plasma and allowed for the metabolic wastes to diffuse easily from the cells of the organ. These were removed by tubing, which followed the same pathway as the blood with one notable difference. At the point that the blood deviated into the entrance of the reservoir's oxygenator, the plasma fluid entered into an artificial kidney, where all the wastes were removed through a dialysis machine and it was then re-turned to the system. From what Sharon saw, she could not discern any difference in the artificial dialysis from the dialy-sis used in hospitalized patients.

There was something different about this balloon though—she moved in for a closer look. "I don't believe it!" she cried. "These are kidneys!" She ran up the row and peered closely at each balloon. They were all housing kidneys in various stages of growth. Now she noticed a small card at the base of each balloon. Up till now, she hadn't been aware of it because her attention had been directed to the contents of each balloon and not on anything else. She read the card. It contained dates and weird hieroglyphics. "Are the kidneys cloned in the same way the livers are?" she asked.

"Yes, they are."

"I assume the codes listed on the identifying cards are genetic then," she said in a smug manner.

"You may assume that."

She was trying to get further information about the pro-cess by which the organs were cloned and grown, but was un-successful in her eager attempt. Both Cook and Matson were remaining extremely closed-mouthed. She was surprised that Barry hardly asked a question, but there was an explanation for her observation. What she didn't know was that Barry had been through this tour a few years ago when he was also in her position. Genome and Bently had enlisted Barry's aid by convincing him of the fortune he would receive from his par-ticipation, which was definitely not the same route by which they were now attempting to gain Sharon's acceptance. She decided not to push the issue and instead walked to the final row of balloons. Quickly, she went to the first one. Sharon stared at a human heart beating in rhythmic fashion, driven to the repetitive contraction that was inherent in all heart muscle. This was almost too much to bear. She shouted at Barry, "Come over here, you won't believe this." Looking around, she saw him standing next to Cook and Matson in idle conversation. She couldn't believe he was so uninterested in it all.

"What have you got?" he asked in a voice that seemed to Sharon to convey a sense of artificiality. He approached her and seemed to act strangely, and Sharon was acutely aware of it. "Look at these hearts! Some also have the lungs attached!"

"That is unbelievable," he said. "This place is really amazing." He was trying hard to show surprise at everything, but he was failing miserably at it, and he sensed that he was. Sharon was acutely aware that Barry's behavior was disingenuous, but she had no idea why.

Barry had always found it hard to hide his feelings, and therefore, it was too difficult a task for him to appear as though this were his first exposure to the lab. After all, he had known about it for a few years now and, to him, it was no big deal. Sharon was excited to a point of exhilaration. In her mind, she ran the multitude of possibilities for mankind. She saw the benefits to humanity that could now become a reality. People could have organ transplants without the fear of missing out on a donor to save their life. The day-to-day existence on the thread of life, never knowing whether your child will be there the next day, was what she saw daily. A relief to parents and adult patients as well, knowing that a new life would be forthcoming and not dependent any longer on a donor supply, was worth everything. She visualized the number of children who would benefit from this, not to mention the millions of adult patients who would be saved from the horrible ordeal of losing a child because there were not enough donors.

She thought about a young man she had cared for some years ago, early in her training, who had contracted hepatitis from a blood transfusion. His liver had failed, and he was confined to a hospital bed where doctors attempted to reverse the ravages of the failing liver with newer drug therapy. They gained slightly in their fight, but each day he sank further into the clutches of irreversible metabolic derangement, and each day a new challenge was presented to the medical staff, how best to buy a few more days in hopes that a donor liver would be available.

Transplant operations were no longer experimental. They were indeed miracles—although the patient exchanged one set of problems for another, the newly acquired problems allowed for a new life. The previous obstacles carried with them a much-reduced longevity. Donated organs to fill the need just weren't available, and there were always as least twice as many patients awaiting organs vs. what was ever available. It had been illegal to pay the families of organ donors since 1984. This law arose out of fear that a black market for organs would develop. After five years, the law was changed to allow for the payment of organs by the private sector, because it was thought that organ transplantation would never be performed in any measurable amounts in private hospitals.

The procedures were so technical that a university hospital would remain "the only game in town."

Sharon smiled to herself. Boy, were they wrong about that one! She had once been told the reason for restricting the state university system, as well as other higher institutions of medical education from purchasing organs, was to keep the academic institutions in line. It was well known that medical school faculty advancement up the academic ladder was directly proportional to the number of scientific papers published in the medical literature. Because this was such a new procedure, it was feared many medical school faculty surgeons might be able to convince the institution to buy organs. Large numbers of surgical cases were needed in order to publish a meaningful article. The large patient base was required for statistical confirmation in evaluation of the surgical outcomes. In any new field of endeavor, there was always a rush for the development of newer techniques, and this was just as true in the field of surgery. Once the development of the surgical techniques was found to be safe, the field of transplantation surgery mushroomed, and surgeons found themselves associating with private hospitals because they were able to procure many more donor organs. Sharon felt so much more alive and grateful that she was able to participate in this process, but it seemed to her that her own talents were dwarfed by what she was currently witnessing. Cook and Matson had just been elevated to the top rung of her ladder. No, they were now saints in her eyes. These men would be responsible for the saving of millions of lives around the world because of their never-ending dedication to the science of genetics. She was deeply awestruck, so much so that she became speechless. Wanting desperately to savor her pleasure and exhilaration, she remained silent and allowed all the good thoughts to bathe her neurons. She reasoned her emotional summit had been the result of internal brain endorphin release, although she had no idea how it had been produced. This was another new area of research that was about to break through the knowledge barrier and give rise to concepts that would stimulate more research of the central nervous system. This, no doubt, would supply answers to the enigma of depression.

She recalled only too vividly her own deep dark depressions of yesteryear and realized well how real it was. It was such a common illness, one might have thought a cure would have been found by now. That was not the case, unfortunately, but it amazed her that genetics had advanced to the point that organs could be cloned, yet depression was still out there ready to pounce on the unwary and plunge them into an abyss. Sharon caught herself and wondered why she was even thinking about it at all, then shook her head, realizing that she was daydreaming.

She walked down the row of hearts, and at the tenth balloon stopped and moved closer. "Oh my dear God in heaven!" she muttered aloud as she bent over closer to the balloon and studied it intensely. What she saw transmitted fear into her own heart. She felt as though she were watching a science fiction movie. Apprehension tried to intimidate her into walking away, but her driving curiosity immediately overcame it, and as bizarre as the object appeared within the confines of the balloon with its dangling tubes, she suppressed her anxiety.

"Dr. Cook, this I do not comprehend!" she exclaimed with conviction. Cook and Matson approached her. "This is an arm, only seven or eight inches long, but still an anatomically intact extremity. From the fingers to the shoulder it is a perfect upper extremity, with blood running from the shoulder vessels just like the liver, kidney, and heart. A normal extremity!" And then it all made sense, first in a blur as pieces of a jigsaw puzzle began to perfectly fit, and then it crystallized flawlessly. "Linda Korn! Barry, that was the third operation? You gave her a brand new extremity, but dared not record any of it because it was still in a research mode without FDA approval. Right?" Her heart was pounding. The adrenalin surge was powerful, and she couldn't stop talking. "This is incredible. It's like a surrealistic dream. But how did—"

Matson interjected, "I believe we have finally arrived at the point where we should return to the conference room and continue where we left off. Please follow me."

Sharon found her mouth open again, accompanied by a look of disbelief as she nodded to Dr. Matson in agreement. Moments later, they were once more in the conference room. Sharon was still in a state of disbelief. She was sure she was dreaming and was awaiting the exodus of the dream, but it never happened.

"Well Dr. Dell, now you have it." Sharon was startled from her trance-like state and jumped at the sound of Cook's voice. Pulling herself together, she tried not to sound like a teenage girl who was overcome by being in the presence of some famous Hollywood actor.

"What a gift you and Dr. Matson have given the world.

Millions will benefit from your research Surely this will net you both the Nobel Prize. I am so honored to have met you both and to have shared in actually seeing the results. What a boon to humanity."

"Dr. Dell, we both are so pleased you see the potential of our research and do so appreciate your very kind words of praise," answered Cook, smiling at Matson as well as Barry.

"Doctor," added Matson quickly, "I would like to try to explain some of the intricacies further at this time, if I may?"

"Yes, please do. I am awaiting it eagerly!" "First, I'll explain how we clone the organs and the extremities. Oh, by the way, we have also cloned lower extremities, as well as intestines and pancreases. Currently, we are writing a protocol for the use of cloned pancreases in insulin-dependent diabetics, which I am sure you would find fascinating, since we will be dealing primarily with the pediatric age group. As you well know, if we could replace the pancreas of a diabetic child with a new transplant, all the complications and ravages of the disease could be avoided. We have a major problem to overcome first in this area though. You'll understand as I explain further.

We have identified the specific genes that control the development of organs and extremities. First, we obtain a bone marrow sample of undifferentiated stem cells from the prospective organ recipient and subject it to extensive genetic DNA study. Here we identify the genetic code of the cell and are able to determine the exons, or coding segments of the DNA. Once we feed this information into our computers, we obtain a map, which identifies upon which chromosome the gene we are looking for is located. We also produce the type O Rh negative red blood cells to perfuse the organs by tissue culture.

"As we have already told you, now we have identified the location of the genes that code for the development of various organs. In addition, we have been able to identify the molecular mechanism that controls the cell cycle. Cell division is a basic property of all life. The development of an organism requires a definitive pattern of cell division, where some cell types divide more often than others, but these divisions all occur at the right times. The genes that control this cell cycle have now been found; the ones that control cell division are of two types. There are those that control cellular metabolism and enlargement, and those that coordinate enlargement and division. Now we have the specific genes that encode the blueprint for a specific organ, and others that will dictate the development of body appendages.

"Here's the way we clone organs. A bone marrow aspiration from the patient requiring an organ transplant is used to obtain a source of undifferentiated hematopoietic stem cells. The genes responsible for cell division and growth are switched on by the addition of activator proteins, which enhance the expression of the gene of interest, thereby increasing the rate of growth one hundred fold. "The cells are grown in a tissue culture until the organ reaches a size that allows us to cannulate the arteries and veins. We then connect the organ to the tubing coming from the oxygenator. The organ remains suspended inside the balloon, surrounded by plasma, as you saw upstairs in the *garden* where all its growing nutrients are supplied. Due to our ability to increase the growth rate, a mature organ may be available for transplant as early as forty days. A child's organ may take only twenty days or so until it is ready for transplant. In the case of an extremity, we do the same basic procedure after we trick the cells into believing they are still part of the entire organism. If the cell were aware that it had been detached from the rest of the developing organism, it would self destruct. That part was a problem for us, but we overcame it eventually by developing a glycoprotein that mimics the glycoprotein on the cells of the native appendages. This protein is added to the nutrients bathing the developing appendage, which is fooled into believing it is still part of the entire organism.

"Now you have it all. Our problem is to figure out why the rejection occurs after two years. We think it may have something to do with our genetic-engineering process, which allows the recipient's body to identify its own cloned organ as foreign. That is why we have to treat the patient with KZ67 for two years."

Sharon was bewildered, yet still euphoric over the vast possibilities for the saving of lives that she would participate in. "I am speechless," she said. The next words she spoke were tempered with reality. "Have you submitted any of this to the FDA for approval?"

"Dr. Dell, we have not, because there wasn't enough substantial data that was acceptable to the FDA," replied Matson.

"Surely these breakthroughs would be acceptable to them!"

"While that might be so, we didn't have enough controlled

data to support the hypothesis of a genetically engineered or cloned organ residing in a host over a period of time. These take years to accumulate."

"What would happen if you were to now report the data collected over the last few years?"

"I'm afraid we dare not do that. It would open a can of worms. Remember, we are also working on the hepatitis virus. We can't take any chances that our work might be curtailed in any way. Our plan is to release our anti-rejection drug KZ67 to the European market very soon. Hopefully, this will be followed by the release of the hepatitis vaccine, and then we will be ready to release cloned organs to the rest of the world. The pressure brought to bear upon the FDA for quick approval will open the U.S.A. market for us as well."

"It is so unfortunate you had to go this route rather than initially obtaining FDA approval but then again, I'm not surprised, since it would have set you back a few years."

"Try about six years at least. The FDA is so stringent in their requirements that we could never have been close to this point five years from now."

"Have there been any fatalities as a result of the clinical experimentation in either organ transplant problems or in rejections, other than the two I am aware of?"

"There have been about a half dozen rejections, all of which I might add were successfully dealt with. A few other minor reactions, but no deaths. Our main thrust now is to continue the clinical trials with KZ67. We now feel that after it is discontinued, steroids should be continued for another year before they are tapered off; however, we need more data to support our theory. If we are right, there will be no further episodes of KZ67 drug-induced hepatitis."

"Alright, now I see it! KZ67 had the ability in some patients to cause toxicity to the liver."

"Yes," answered Matson, "now you can understand what happened to Linda Korn. She was given KZ67 after her upper extremity transplant to prevent rejection of the extremity. Her results were perfect, but she developed liver toxicity from it, which led to liver failure and the need for a transplant."

"Dr. Dell," interrupted Cook, "will you help us in our effort to complete the research project?"

"What do you want of me, Dr. Cook?" she asked innocently.

"We want you to continue performing transplants. As you are aware, we are expected to get hit hard with the new hepatitis virus, and the anticipation is a tenfold increase in the need for liver transplants. Secondly, we want to feel that our secret is safe with you." "You are doing something that is not approved by a regulatory agency. My concern is for the kids and adults whose lives will be saved through your efforts. Your secret is safe, but I hope you will at least consider the possibility of talking with the FDA in generalities, and maybe there is a way to make it all legal. Right now, in the USA alone, there are at least thirty thousand deaths a year from lack of a donor organ, and more to be expected with the new hepatitis virus. God knows how many people might die worldwide in addition if your work isn't completed."

Both Cook and Matson walked to her and extended their hands. Barry also offered his hand, which she accepted as well.

Sharon had the feeling deep down that she might regret her decision. What real choices did she have? That it was not an approved method and might be fraught with problems that would be a health hazard? Organs were supplied by a different method, that was all. *What's the big deal? The big deal is it's dishonest and unethical!* She thought she heard a small voice add the last thought.

Almost four hours had passed, and Sharon was mentally fatigued. She was famished and was grateful when Cook announced that lunch was to be served in five minutes. They had arranged for lunch to be delivered in the conference room. Sharon had many questions for Barry and would have easily forgone lunch here in deference to a Big Mac. For her, that was an extreme sacrifice in view of the fact that she loathed fast food, but she really had no choice. but lunch arrived, and to her surprise, two other well-dressed gentlemen arrived just before it was served.

— 14 —

GETTING DOWN
TO BUSINESS

"**D**r. Dell, I would like to introduce you to Mr. Michael Rome, CEO of Genome Corporation," said Cook. "He is my boss." Rome extended an outstretched hand, which Sharon accepted with a smile.

"I am delighted to make your acquaintance, sir."

He nodded gratefully and looked toward Malkin. "Dr. Dell, this is David Malkin, CEO of Bently Drug Company." Promptly, the other man offered his greeting to her in an officious manner. Both CEOs shook hands with Barry, and Sharon overheard one of them whisper, "How did it go?"

Lunch arrived, and they all sat at the long conference table. Chicken sandwiches on focaccia bread with roasted red peppers, brushed with a tangy dressing that was served with iced cappuccino coffee and an assortment of cookies. After the small talk, which largely centered about Sharon, Malkin asked Sharon how she had enjoyed the visit to the research lab.

"The most fascinating I have ever seen, to say the least. It was like a trip into space!"

"We are delighted you feel that way, Dr. Dell. I'm confidant we can count on your support then?" asked Malkin, pushing hard for an affirmative answer.

Sharon became suddenly aware of the pressure. What indeed did he mean by support? His demeanor suggested he meant more than the simple question implied. Suddenly, she was gripped with deep suspicion. Was she doing the correct thing in this complicated situation? Something deep down was gnawing at her, and she began to identify the feeling as similar to those she'd had when she was an intern on the pediatric service. Why was she starting to feel the pangs of guilt? She had done nothing wrong!

Her mind raced through the morning's experiences which were still vivid. *Oh yes*, she said to herself, *Doctors Cook and Matson both used the same phraseology. They asked if they could depend on me, and I felt as odd then as I do now.* Quickly, she drew rationalization from her depths and answered the question. "You can count on my support for your project. It will benefit humanity greatly, and I am proud to be able to offer my small part."

"Not only will it benefit humanity, but it will benefit our stockholders as well," stated Michael Rome with pride. He cast an imperceptible glance at David Malkin, who remained still.

"Maybe now Dr. Dell will be able to transplant the patients who were scheduled at Squire in San Diego," said Malkin.

"What patients are you referring to?" she asked with a hint of caution. Malkin looked at Barry pleadingly, and he got the message. "Ah … Sharon, there was a recent investigation by the DOC at Squire, and they are currently nosing around trying to get information on our transplant patients."

Sharon looked stunned. "What kind of information do they want?"

"Evidently, one of their inspectors found in his audit that transplant patients arriving for a second transplant were not taking any anti-rejection drugs, and they became alarmed by this. They think that the patients were receiving substandard medical care and have obtained a temporary restraining order on the hospital until they investigate further."

Sharon was astonished. "Why weren't they made aware of the research protocol?" she inquired innocently.

"All the patients belong to the World Health Care HMO. If it were discovered that clinical research was going on without FDA approval, all hell would break loose. They would come down heavily on World Health Care for using nonapproved methods of therapy. They could even lose their license to sell health coverage in California," interjected Rome. "We need their help in this research also."

"I don't follow you," she said.

"World Health Care is a partner in our research. They were delighted to allow clinical testing on their patients because, in return, they will derive financial benefit when we release the hepatitis vaccine."

"You mean that the potential cost savings from a lower liver transplant rate will increase their profit?"

"Well, that is another way of looking at it, I suppose," answered Rome.

"And these transplant patients can only be operated on at TWMC?" asked Sharon.

"You see, Dr. Dell, World Health Care has a tertiary contract for high-level care with Squire and TWMC only."

"That answers a question that has bothered me for a long time. I wondered why we were doing so many transplants at TWMC."

"We have no choice in the matter, Sharon," said Barry. "There are twenty or so already on the list and scheduled. Their organs have been growing and are awaiting each patient."

"How many children?" asked Sharon.

"I think at last count about ten."

Dr. Cook, who had sat silent up to now, chimed in. "Don't forget the hepatitis epidemic. There will be many more transplant patients over the next twelve months."

"I will do my part to further the gathering of information for the project. Right now, though, I am going to be late for my clinic." She looked at her watch and stood up. The room resonated as the five gentlemen also stood and pushed back their chairs from the table. They were accompanied by a security guard to the car.

– 15 –

LEGALITY CONFIRMED

Sharon was engrossed in her daily activities of running her department, teaching residents, and performing surgery. In addition, she was in charge of the twice-weekly transplant clinic, where it seemed there was an increased and never-ending supply of potential patients. She was in her office on Thursday afternoon when she received a telephone call from her father.

"Hi Dad, where have you been?" she asked him, as though she were interrogating a child who was late for dinner.

"I've been out of town for two weeks. The DOC had me doing audits on hospitals in Fresno, Bakersfield, and San Diego. I just returned yesterday."

When Sharon heard San Diego, her heart took a leap. She felt a sense of panic as she prayed that her Dad was not the one who'd found the problem at Squire. "Well, did you meet any available women?" she cajoled him.

"No, I was too busy," he answered with a laugh. "That reminds me Sharon, I want to ask your professional opinion about something."

Sharon winced. "Of course, what about, Dad?" She felt like disconnecting the phone at that point, because her intuition told her what was coming.

"Sharon, are all transplant patients required to be taking anti-rejection drugs?"

There it was. He had been the one who audited Squire. "Ah, why are you asking?"

"In my audit of Squire Hospital in San Diego, I noted that patients coming there for second transplants were not on any specific regime of anti-rejection drug therapy and I thought that it was odd."

She hesitated. If she lied to him, he would easily find out that these patients were required to take these drugs for life. On the other hand, if she disclosed the truth to him about KZ67, she would have to inform him that the drug was not FDA-approved. Even more of a concern was that initially it had been thought it could be discontinued after two years, only for it to be eventually discovered that that was a grave error. The newest ideas were that prednisone should be continued for another year before discontinuation of the steroid completely.

"Sharon, did you hear my question?" "Yes, Dad. Presently, all patients must be kept on anti-rejection therapy for life. Steroids are often able to be discontinued though." She bit down hard on her lower lip. She wanted desperately to tell him that the drug had now been modified and soon it could be stopped after two years. Sharon knew he would be obliged by his own sense of ethics and morals to report it to the State Department of Corporations, who would move in quickly to shut the program down. She didn't remember the last time she had lied to her father, and it grieved her now that she was considering it at all. If she told him the truth, the lives of thousands of children and adults would be lost because the cloned organs wouldn't be available. How could she allow that to happen? One lie would save all those lives, but to tell the truth would snuff them all out. And then there was the onslaught of the hepatitis epidemic and the children's lives that couldn't be saved for the lack of donor organs. What was just as bad was that she didn't know how she would be able to cope with lying to her father. Their relationship had always been one of mutual honesty and trust. This made her the most sad in the moment—the violation of his trust.

"Okay, that's what I thought, but these patients weren't getting any, and I think that somebody dropped the ball and that's why they had rejection and the need for a new organ transplant. What do you think?"

She was in a difficult spot now. One lie was too much, and now she was placed in a position of having to pass judgment on her colleagues. "Dad, I've got to go. My pager is going off. I have to do an emergency transplant right now. I'll call you later!" She tried to put just the right amount of inflection in her voice to emphasize the urgency of the matter, and desperately hoped it would work.

"Call me when you can. I love you."

Sharon hung up the phone and rubbed her forehead, then went to the kitchen and heated a kettle of water on the stove for tea. She needed to rethink the entire situation again because she didn't feel good about her position. Way down deep, she knew the reason.

The next day, she became more anxious over the fact that she was now involved in something that just didn't sit right with her. She picked up the phone.

"Mr. Foxworthy, this is Dr. Dell. Do you have a moment?"

"Certainly, what can I do for you?"

"Well it's a long story, but I would like to discuss something with the hospital's attorney."

"May I ask what it concerns?"

"I'd rather not say at this time. Let's just say it concerns a possible ethical question."

"Does it involve TWMC?"

"I'm afraid it does. I would feel a lot better if I could discuss it with the hospital's attorneys, since they do represent TWMC interests."

"I'll have my secretary call our attorneys, and they'll call you to set up an appointment."

"That would be fine. Could you ask them to call me today? I want to get this settled as soon as possible."

"It would be my pleasure." He immediately placed a call to the hospital attorney, Mr. Andrew Barotta.

"Andy, this is James Foxworthy. I have just been asked by one of our physicians, Dr. Dell, to contact you and ask that you call her back today. She has an ethical problem of sorts that she wishes to talk to you about."

"Do you have any idea what it is about?"

"My gut reaction is that she is getting cold feet about the research at the laboratories. She is one of our transplant surgeons, and yesterday she was given the grand tour."

"Fine. I will see her today and soothe her feathers."

Barotta hung up and called his secretary. "Anne, please call Dr. Dell at TWMC and see if I can meet with her later this afternoon."

"I'm on it right now, Mr. Barotta."

A few minutes later, Dr. Dell had agreed to meet him at his office that afternoon.

It was shortly after 4 p.m. when Sharon entered Barotta's office. The office was located in the East Tower of the Century City office complex on the twenty-sixth floor. She was duly impressed with the office as she looked around while waiting for Barotta. Plush carpets of royal blue adorned the floors, and the blue-gray couch she was sitting on was made of Italian plush leather. She smiled at the secretary, who was busy answering the flood of calls while attempting to work at her computer.

Andrew Barotta introduced himself as he walked into the waiting room.

"So good of you to drive all the way to see me, Dr. Dell." He extended his hand and helped her from the couch. "Please, follow me."

He led her into his private office. It looked out upon the Century City Hotel as well as Santa Monica Blvd. Pigeons were flying nearby, trying to land on the windowsill, but were precluded from doing so by the presence of large, slender nails sticking into the air about four inches. Some seemed to hover with outspread wings staring directly at her, no doubt hoping she would open the window so they could land safely.

Sharon seated herself in the chair situated directly in front of his massive desk. The entire top of the desk was clad in red inlaid leather and barren of any work product, which made her wonder how busy he was, since she gauged productivity by the amount of paperwork piled on her desk.

"How may I help you, Dr. Dell?" asked Barotta.

"Mr. Barotta, I want your advice on an issue which is bothering me. Are you familiar with the Research Laboratory in Malibu?"

"Well, yes I am. It is a joint venture between Genome Corporation and World Health Care."

"So you are aware that TWMC receives its *donor* organs from them?"

"Yes, I am."

"My concern is that I was asked to support their research and efforts."

"What was meant by support?"

"That's just it. They never said anything other than they wanted me to keep doing transplant surgery at TWMC, even though I now know how the organs are made."

"You mean the cloning of the organs?"

"Exactly. I feel somewhat concerned about it since it is not yet an FDA-approved method."

"I really wouldn't let that bother you, Doctor. Your involvement is entirely from the clinical side. The organ procurement is the responsibility of TWMC. Look at it the same way you would if the organs were bought rather than donated. The method of procurement is the sole responsibility of TWMC, and you have no liability at all."

"I just have a problem with accepting it because it is so foreign to me."

"I'll tell you what, Doctor, I will prepare a hold harmless release for you. Will that suffice?"

"What is that?"

"A hold harmless is a legal document which states that the grantor, in this case TWMC, agrees to accept total responsibility for the organs, and should anyone sue you personally, they would stand behind you completely. TWMC would pay for your defense and pay any and all judgments which might come about as a result of such a suit. In California, you know, anything can happen."

"That would sure make me feel a lot better about it." She thought about his offer again. If this were not legal, TWMC would not be making this proposal to her. "Dr. Dell, FDA approval is not necessary for us in order to use the cloned organs, because we are a teaching hospital. We are exempt from it. The same way that we are exempt from being sued by a plaintiff who alleges that an experimental drug caused harm. Our doctors administer these drugs all the time, and all the patients sign specific medical releases, just like they do for the donor transplant organs."

"Oh, I didn't know that the patients sign medical releases for the organs. I've only seen the general release for treatment and surgery."

"That is because the organ release for liability is obtained through informed consent by this office. Each patient is shown a twenty-minute video tape, which is generic and explains all the risks and other options open to the patient. Dr. Swenz then speaks with each patient and obtains a witnessed signature. This is followed by a letter from my office reiterating the risks and asking the patient to again certify by their signature that they are willing to go through with the transplant procedure."

"That sounds great. I feel better already."

"Dr. Dell, we have been doing this for many years now and have never had a problem. Patients are very happy to have their diseases cured, so to speak, and usually at no expense to them since the HMO pays all the costs."

"I am satisfied, Mr. Barotta. Please send the hold harmless agreements to me at TWMC."

"I will have them in your hands within a week. Thank you for coming by."

Sharon left the office and felt lighter, as though a weight had been lifted from her. She was now convinced that she could continue the transplants without worry, but she didn't know TWMC was also a financial part of the joint venture partnership and Barotta was therefore somewhat biased in his opinion. As far as she knew, Barotta was only the hospital's attorney, whose sole function was to make certain TWMC dealings were all legal and proper.

Back in the office, Barotta picked up his phone. "Hello James, this is Andrew. I have convinced the good doctor that all is well. She will be no problem to you."

"Great Andy, send me your bill—and oh, why don't you bill us for an additional thirty hours of fees at your usual $300 an hour. I will approve payment upon receipt."

"The bill will be in the mail tomorrow, and thank you for your kindness, James."

Sharon returned to TWMC and buried herself in her

work. She loathed having free time, because it gave her opportunity to think, and this caused her anxiety. That week, the local press gave legitimacy to the hepatitis epidemic that had now arrived in the U.S. As luck would have it, the outbreak occurred first in Los Angeles and was tracked to a group of Asians who'd arrived in the city on tour five months before. The U.S. Health Department had tracked the tour throughout California and Hawaii. At every major tourist attraction, an outbreak of hepatitis was identified, and many of the fast food restaurants were among the hardest hit. Those infected by the tourists unknowingly passed the virus along to innocent Californians, who'd begun to reveal evidence of the disease over the last two weeks. Reports from the medical community made to the various county health departments had shown an attack rate of epidemic proportions. Sharon calculated in her mind that this would result in numerous cases of refractory liver failure within a month or so. Many of these cases would result in the need for transplant surgery, but she felt confident that the need would be met with success at TWMC. The only problem was that the only patients who had a real chance at getting a "donor" liver available on time were those patients who belonged to World Health Care HMO. She felt much better now that she had been informed of the epidemic—almost as though it vindicated her decision to guard the secret.

Standing in the cafeteria line at TWMC, she was deep in thought when a physician asked her if he might pass her in the line.

"Oh, I am so sorry. I guess I was daydreaming. Please

excuse me. She allowed him to pass and then retrieved a sandwich from the shelf along with a cup of coffee. Leaving the cashier, she looked around for an empty chair. The noon hour was exceptionally crowded, and Sharon had almost given up, when the same doctor approached her.

"Hi, I'm Mike Herbert—will you join me?" He gestured toward his table.

"Thank you, I appreciate the offer. By the way, I'm Sharon Dell."

When they were seated, Mike asked, "What is your specialty?"

"I'm a transplant surgeon. What is your expertise?"

"I am an oncologist." She munched some of her sandwich and was acutely aware of Mike's interest in her. She felt flattered and kind of liked his attention. Mike asked her how long she had been at TWMC and made small talk for the next forty-five minutes. Sharon found herself attracted to his good looks and sense of humor. Unknown to her, he had the same feelings.

"Well, I've got to run to my clinic. Do you eat at this time every day?"

Without hesitation, she answered, "Yes, I usually do."

"Great, maybe next time you'll save me a seat." He gave her a broad smile and walked away, leaving her alone, sipping her cup of coffee.

The next six weeks at TWMC were hectic. She was evaluating increased numbers of patients in the clinic who were in need of livers, and almost two-thirds of them were children.

– 16 –

A Weekend in Vegas

B arry was looking forward to the weekend. He was still feeling somewhat uneasy about the visit to the research lab with Sharon. She appeared to have accepted the program, but he still wasn't certain, and his financial future rested on the completion of the research projects. The timely arrival of the vaccine and acceptance of cloned organs throughout the world, not withstanding the U.S.'s FDA approval, was at stake. Barry drove home, packed his small bag, and drove to LAX to catch the seven o'clock flight to Las Vegas. He didn't want to miss the flight, because the consequences would be disastrous.

Sitting back in his reclining seat, he thought about the problem at hand. He had been coming to Vegas for years and usually made the trip twice a month, at least until recently. He thought about his childhood growing up in a small, provincial town in Rhode Island where life was drab, and how he had lived for the day he could leave the state. After four years, he'd matriculated with a B.S. degree at the University of Rhode Island and moved to New Jersey, where he commuted to medical school in New York City.

He had been poor and had to work his way through school as a laboratory technician in a local county hospital in Bergen County. There, he worked a few nights each week, as well as weekends, in order to earn enough money to exist and pay tuition. Many a night he was awoken and had to drive to the hospital to perform laboratory tests on a patient. The next day in school, he would be exhausted and find himself falling asleep throughout the day. Sometimes it was more than he could bear. He longed for the end of the grueling pressure of maintaining the passing grades required for graduation from medical school.

He had been fortunate enough to receive the benefits of the G.I. Bill after his discharge from the U.S. Navy. It paid his rent but left only fifty dollars each month for the purchase of the George Washington Bridge commuter tickets. A 1956 Studebaker was his mode of transportation, which always seemed to be enshrouded in a cloud of black smoke, unless it was parked. A book of ten tickets purchased weekly for ten dollars was a lot of money in 1965, he thought to himself with a laugh.

Barry tried to cast these thoughts from his mind, but found it too difficult. Wondering why he had been thinking about his past, he then attempted to fall asleep but was unable to do that either. Suddenly, he sat upright and sipped the coffee brought by the flight attendant, savoring the warm liquid as it caressed his mouth. He felt very uneasy when the attendant told him they would be landing in twenty-five minutes. His story needed to be straight when he met with Adrian. *How did I allow this to happen to me?* All his life, he had been poor and never had available money for even the smallest of luxuries. He'd arrived in California in 1970 to begin his orthopedics residency at LA Children's Hospital. Two weeks after he started, he met her.

She was tempting and alluring, and provoked an immense sense of well-being in his soul. The meetings became more frequent as the years ensued but finally reached the point where it was completely out of control. No matter how hard he tried, he couldn't let her go. She latched on to him with the tenacity of super glue and never gave up the position she occupied in his life. Now he would have to pay for his indiscretions. The price, he feared, would no doubt be high. He loved the game, the chase and the excitement she instilled in him. He couldn't break off the relationship no matter how hard he tried, and always returned only to be abused by her again. It was too bad he had never met a lady that held his interest other than the one he was so infatuated with, but that was his determined lot. He was a victim. She was his Lady Luck, but he still couldn't admit to his gambling addiction.

The plane landed and he disembarked, carrying his small overnight bag, then went to the front of the airport where he hailed a cab. He checked into the Conquistador and placed a call to Adrian, who promised he would be there in twenty minutes.

More sweat time, he thought, as he mixed himself a drink from the mini-bar. He sat back and waited for Adrian's arrival, dreading the knock that came much too soon. Adrian entered and shook hands with Barry.

"Well, how was the trip this time, Doc?" asked Adrian.

"Not bad. I'm back to try again, and this time I brought ten thousand dollars to help me recoup my losses."

"How much did you bring for me?"

"Look, I know that I owe you thirty thousand dollars, but I have always paid you everything, haven't I? I need some more time to get you caught up. I have ten thousand for you now, and if I'm lucky tonight and tomorrow, I might be able to give you at least another ten thousand dollars before I leave on Sunday."

"Doc, you know that I've worked with you, and over the past five years, I've let you go for weeks, but I can't do it anymore. The new owners of the casino are on my back and I got to produce or it's my neck. I already went out on a limb for you and extended your note six weeks. I can't go any longer. This debt has got to be paid now, or it's out of my hands. The boss expects the cash today!"

Barry's heart skipped a beat when he heard the words *it's out of my hands*. He knew only too well what that could mean. A friend of his had once told him about the time the boys from Vegas had paid a visit to collect on a much smaller debt and he was unable to pay the money. They' threatened to have his wrists broken if he didn't pay in a week's time. They returned as promised one week later for the payment, but John had miraculously found the money. They also made him pay an extra fifteen hundred dollars, which the boys explained was their fee for *collecting* the debt.

His hands were his work. He was a gifted surgeon and could not afford an accident that would prevent him from entering the operating room. "Alright, here's twenty thousand now, and I will write you a check for the balance." He withdrew a small check from his wallet, imprinted with the Bank of America logo. He had a ten-thousand-dollar line of cash credit, which was tied to his credit card. He had never used it before and was very happy that he had it available.

"Thanks, Doc. Now that you are even, I can extend you a five-thousand-dollar credit for chips with the understanding it will be repaid within two weeks at the usual twenty-five percent interest rate." He handed a slip of paper to Barry, who quickly handed it back to his long-time friend. He was going to quit gambling forever.

"Well, Doc, if you change your mind, give me a call and I'll notify the pit boss to accept your marker." He left Barry to himself and shut the door quietly. Barry threw himself on the bed and switched on TV using the remote. The screen exploded with vibrant color containing the following message: "For our very special guests to whom we would like to show our appreciation, enter your personal four-digit code." This was the very latest in personal TV communication that had been installed recently in the Conquistador Hotel by the new owners. A bank of rooms were always reserved for the high rollers at the casino. Experience showed that the majority of these men were easily lured back by the *special favors* supplied by the house in the form of a surprise. In the past, this was accomplished by the management arranging for a girl to go directly to the room of its guest. On occasion, it proved to be disastrous when the guest already had a female companion. So as not to cause any embarrassment, they provided for this—for each special guest who had been assigned a room within the reserved bank of rooms—by using a specially installed menu on the TV. The menu selection was such that it enabled the girl to know in advance all the pleasures which the viewer preferred. It was an ingenious method that removed any inhibitions from the viewer by alerting the girl in advance to his likes and dislikes. Barry had availed himself of this once before.

I'm certainly not going to the casino, he thought as he entered his code. The screen changed, now showing the head shots of twelve women. Each photo was numbered and the instructions called for a numerical selection for a better look at the product. Barry entered his choice and the next screen disclosed further poses with the models wearing various apparel. Another selection allowed for the inspection of the girl in provocative poses without clothes. The next selection process called for a choice as to how the meeting should occur. One might choose to have an intimate descriptive phone call first followed by a room visit and finally the viewer was asked to rate and select the various sexual positions and acts that were a turn on for him.

The girl arrived at the room in ten minutes and marched through the script that Barry had directed through his selections.

It was 3 a.m. when he woke to find that his bed partner gone. *I can't blame her—she makes her living by* piece *work*. He laughed aloud at his double entendre and felt again the familiar urge for the excitement of the tables. Knowing that it was all happening just five floors below was more than he could bear. Rationalizing to himself that this was the last time he would ever be in Las Vegas and he only had one thousand dollars in his wallet, he quickly dressed and marched out the door. His heart was beating fast in anticipation of the casino with its throngs gathered at various tables. He might even win twenty thousand dollars in a few short hours, but then, he was only going to spend a thousand, and he could well afford that much.

– 17 –

THE AUDIT
FROM DELL

Another two weeks rapidly passed without Sharon's no-
ticing. She was entrenched in her work and refused to
give any further thought to the Research Laboratory. She was
in the business of restoring lives, and that was all that really
mattered.

Monday morning at 9 a.m., a middle-aged, well-dressed
gentleman carrying a brown briefcase walked through the
front door of TWMC and asked for the hospital administrator's office. He was directed to Mr. James Foxworthy's office
by one of the volunteers. Walking up to the desk of the secretary, he gave her his card and waited while she called her
boss to announce the arrival of Karl Dell, M.D., from the
Department of Corporations. In seconds, James Foxworthy
appeared at his office door and approached Karl with his
right hand extended, in anticipation of a greeting.

"I am happy to make your acquaintance, Doctor," said
Foxworthy.

"Thank you, sir. May we speak in private?"

Foxworthy led Karl into the office and shut the door, then walked to his desk and sat down.

"May I offer you coffee or tea?" he asked in his most congenial manner.

"Thank you, but I am coffee'd out," answered Karl, smiling pleasantly.

"Very well, Doctor. what can I do for you?"

"Mr. Foxworthy, the DOC has sent me here to do an on-site audit." He reached over and unlocked his briefcase, from which he retrieved a document and handed it to the CEO.

Foxworthy quickly scanned it and was visibly shaken.

Karl continued, "This is a Subpoena Duces Tecums issued by the Attorney General's Office for all hospital and clinic records of all World Health Care HMO surgical transplant patients performed in this hospital over the last five years."

"What is this all about?" asked Foxworthy, trying to appear nonchalant despite the beginning of a visual aura that heralded the start of a migraine.

"The DOC wants to review all these records. Copies can be made while I begin to review some of them today. We are looking for answers to some medical quality of care issues."

"What type of issues would that be?"

"We have found after auditing another facility in San Diego that patients who required a second organ transplant have not been receiving any anti-rejection drug therapy. We feel, perhaps, the failure to treat them with these drugs led to the rejection process and the eventual need for a second organ transplant. If that is the case, there will be further investigation by the Medical Board of California, which will try to identify the doctors responsible for the treatment of these poor people. It's also apparent that all the patients belong to World Health Care HMO." Foxworthy blanched when he heard the response. He was well aware of the research protocols administered by Barry Swenz under the supervision of Genome and Bently. His heart began to race, and a fine sweat appeared on his forehead. *If they ever find out, we could all go down.* "Well, why don't I take you to our medical records department and they can begin pulling the charts for you," he said in a solicitous manner. He walked to the door and led Karl outside to the large halls of the hospital. They made small talk as they ambled through the lengthy corridors before finally arriving at the medical records department. Foxworthy allowed Karl to enter ahead of him and then asked the young lady at the computer if Mrs. Marcos was in. Lydia Marcos was the hospital's chief medical record director, a very competent and likable woman in her late forties. Her demeanor gained her acceptance by the medical staff and her coworkers. "Lydia, I would like you to meet Doctor, ahh ..." He quickly glanced at the card Karl had given him earlier. "Dell." Then it sank in.

"Dr. Dell, we have a Dr. Sharon Dell here with us, do you know her?"

"I should say so!" responded Karl with admiration and pride exuding in his voice. "She is my daughter."

Foxworthy felt real panic. *Of course, I now understand,* he said to himself. He turned toward Lydia and continued, "Please help the doctor in any way you can. Here is the subpoena for your files." He shook hands with Karl and left the department, almost running all the way back to his office.

"Hold all my calls for the next twenty minutes and see if you can get Dr. Swenz on the telephone for me." A moment later, he was connected to Dr. Barry Swenz.

"Dr. Swenz, I thought you told me everything went well with Dr. Dell's visit at the research lab last month?" he asked suspiciously.

"Why yes, I did. What is the matter?"

"The matter is that, as we speak, we are undergoing a medical audit by the DOC, and guess who served me with the subpoena?"

"I haven't the slightest clue, James. How would I know?"

"Well, you'd better sit down. Dr. Karl Dell, Sharon's father." The line was silent for what felt like an eternity.

"I never knew she had a father who was a physician. What is he looking for?"

"He's looking at the last five years of transplant surgeries, trying to find out why World Health Care HMO patients did not receive anti-rejection drugs after their transplants. He thinks that is what caused those patients to need a second organ transplant. Obviously he doesn't know the real cause was that KZ67 is hepatotoxic."

"My God! If he discovers that I have not continued the KZ67 beyond two years of surgery, I'm in trouble. It may even trigger a focus audit on all the liver transplants that had to be repeated."

"What about the fact that KZ67 isn't FDA approved?"

"Don't add insult to injury, please. I am well aware of

the liability." Barry was feeling panic. The anxiety was over-whelming and his heart fluttered twice while he was hyper-ventilating. He started to feel faint but caught himself and made a conscious effort to hold his breath and restore the proper acid base equilibrium that had gone awry by virtue of his excessive respiratory rate. He suppressed the nausea that accompanied the pins and needles he felt in his face and hands.

"Dr. Swenz, are you still there?"

"Yes, I'm here. Let me get back to you, James—I need some time to think."

He hung up the phone, and for the first time since he had started on the Research Laboratory project, he experienced fear. He dialed the personal number of Michael Rome and brought him up to date on the recent developments.

"I am convinced Sharon is at the root of all this!" he screamed.

"Calm down now, Doctor, and let's look at this rationally. Why do you suspect Sharon?"

"She knows everything about our program. She must have had second thoughts about working with us and keeping the secret, so she told her father. My God, he works for the DOC. What better way to pull the rug from beneath us. He marched in here with a subpoena from the Attorney General's Office. When they audit, they always send a letter and instruct the hospital on what type of data they want. I have never heard of a subpoena for the purposes of an audit."

"Why do you think they did that?"

"Obviously, they wanted to see the actual records

produced and copied. Someone was afraid that the charts might have been *doctored* to reflect the appropriate data they sought."

"That makes sense. What can we do about it now? They will find what they are looking for."

"Yes, and I'm left holding the bag!"

"Please get a grip on yourself. Let me first talk to David Malkin, and we'll get back to you soon."

"Do it fast. We need to deal with that bitch."

Two hours later, Barry was looped into a conference call with Mr. Rome and Mr. Malkin.

"Dr. Swenz, we have discussed this recent crisis at the hospital and wish to offer a few suggestions to you," said Rome.

"Go on. I'm waiting."

"We have a plan that might solve the problem for us all. What would you think Sharon's response might be if her father had liver failure from hepatitis and required a liver transplant?"

"What did you say?" responded Swenz in a loud incredulous manner.

"Just follow me for a moment. Isn't it plausible that if it did happen, she would want to get him a liver fast?"

"Of course she would. So what?" he answered in annoyance.

"Well, we could supply one fast, but Sharon would have to agree to keep her mouth shut about anything she knows as part of the bargain. Do you think her father's life would be impetus enough?"

"Sure, but what stops her from talking after the operation?"

"Our research department has developed a process by which a transplanted organ may have incorporated within it a microchip that activates a code that will cause cells to die. The liver would then die by attrition, because cells could not be replaced, which all organs do throughout life. We have developed a process that can activate this through the use of an electromagnetic force device that causes code process to begin."

"That is truly remarkable, but how does it work on the DNA?" asked Barry in astonishment.

"It's too technical and I don't understand it, but Dr. Cook calls it apoptosis. He can fill you in on the particulars later."

"So, anyone with this transplanted liver may have an induced activation at any time in the future, which will lead to the death of the liver. It's like walking around with a time bomb that can be triggered at any time."

"That's right. That way, we control Sharon, and she'll keep our secret."

"All well and good, but how does Karl Dell get end-stage liver disease?"

"That, my dear doctor, is where we shall perform our part. Trust us, we *will* talk again," answered Rome.

–18–

DOCTOR DELL EXAMINES DOCTOR DELL

It had already been more than a week since Karl had visited TWMC. He had submitted the hospital charts to his supervisor, who in turn locked them in his office filing cabinet. He told Karl there were more pressing matters that concerned the Department of Corporations, and with the personnel cutbacks, further work on TWMC organ transplant cases would have to wait for now. Karl was disappointed, since he was convinced there was incompetence and malpractice at the root of the problem. He was assigned to another more pressing problem relating to another HMO which had numerous complaints filed against it for failure to pay claims in a timely manner. The state was more concerned with insuring prompt payments to medical providers than in the quality of health care provided by the managed care plans. This resulted in political pressure exerted on his boss to devote the time in the financial area rather than the delivery of medical care.

Karl was diligently working at his desk when his phone rang.

"Dr. Dell, this is Dr. Harper of the State Department of Health."

"Yes," interrupted Karl, "I believe you are the assistant director of the department."

"Doctor, the reason I am calling is to inform you of our plans to inoculate all state employees who spend any time in hospitals against the hepatitis epidemic we are currently experiencing. The virus is extremely virulent and may cause liver failure in as little as four to six weeks, and as you may know, the mortality rate is very high. We have received a batch of vaccine from a drug company which we are going to use to immunize those who are at risk. Our broad definition of risk has been determined to be anyone working in or frequently visiting hospitals. We are beginning the immunizations immediately."

"I didn't realize a vaccine was available at this time."

"Oh yes, it is, but only for health care workers. We have not broken the news to the press yet so as not to cause public dissension. That is why we need to get the program underway now. We have designated a number of our nurses to immunize people on the job, such as yourself, who are much too busy to come to a clinic for the vaccine. May I send our nurse over to give you the immunization today?"

"Certainly. I will be here doing paperwork all day." Karl was convinced of the usefulness of immunizations and was delighted that he didn't have to travel to some designated clinic to get the shot. At three o'clock that afternoon, the nurse arrived and administered the shot. It smarted slightly but rapidly dissipated and he returned to the job at hand, manifested by the piles of paper that were assigned to his desk. He had to read volumes of data that had been gathered by the DOC.

Over the next month, Karl could be found each day working at his desk until 6 and occasionally 7 p.m. The days flew by rapidly and there seemed to be no time for Karl's private life. When he got home, he found that it was 9 p.m. by the time he had prepared and eaten dinner. Relaxing with the news roundup pushed the clock to ten. Many evenings he dozed off during the news, and on others, he chatted with friends on the phone, but when he tried to call his daughter, he found she wasn't home. Obviously, she was still at the hospital or had been called back to her job for an emergency. Karl wanted to believe that Sharon had some kind of social life, but he knew too well it wasn't likely. He made a concerted effort to reach her, and after three successive evenings, was finally victorious in his endeavor.

"Sharon, finally I caught you at home. Is everything alright?"

"I am just fine, Dad," she replied, well aware that he was concerned about her physical well-being.

"I have been pretty busy myself at the DOC."

Sharon cringed. She hoped she wouldn't be drawn into a defense argumentative position concerning any medical issues relating to transplant surgeries—especially those performed at TWMC. Her concern was that Barry was responsible for the postoperative care of the patients, which included treatment with anti-rejection medication. The charts lacked the specific recording of this data, and after about two years, all the patients were discharged from follow-up care. She worried that her colleague, Barry, might have to explain his care to an unsympathetic board.

"I assume your audit at TWMC went alright?" she asked, trying to coax a positive answer from her dad.

"I gathered a lot of data but didn't get that deep into it. It was placed on hold by the director of the DOC because of a manpower shortage. There seem to be more pressing needs at this time."

Immediately Sharon felt a burden had been lifted from her very being. *Maybe everything will turn out alright after all.* "How have you been feeling yourself, Dad?"

"Other than the long hours, I'm fine. Just a little tired lately, but I think it's because I haven't been getting my eight hours each night."

"Listen Dad, you don't have to work like that. I am sure they don't expect you to take work home with you every night," said Sharon sternly.

"It's not that, dear—I do all the work at the office, but I can't get out of there until seven or later. By the time I get home, make dinner, and eat, it's already ten o'clock. Then, it's eleven thirty before I go to bed, and I get up at five thirty."

"You have to get your rest. Please promise me that you will leave the job like everyone else at five o'clock," she pleaded.

"You worry too much Sharon, but I will promise."

"We need to get together soon. I'm sorry I didn't see you when you were at TWMC, but I was in surgery all day and most of the evening."

"I know. I checked on you."

"What about next weekend? I could drive up and spend a few days."

"That would be great. So I'll see you in ten days."

"See you then, and by the way Dad, I love you."

"I love you too. Good night."

The next day, Karl noted that he had a spring in his step, and he knew it was because his daughter was coming to visit him soon. He always felt more alive and full of energy whenever Sharon said she was coming to spend a few days with him. He adored his daughter, and more than anything else in the world, he loved to spend quiet time with her. Discussing the recent advances in medicine or recent novels that one of them had read went a long way to uplift his spirit. He returned to his desk and started to review the heaps of data he'd been assigned. That evening, at 5 p.m., he left the office. By the time he got home, he felt more tired than usual but attributed it to "coming down with a cold."

But the following morning he felt awful and was certain he was getting the flu. He ached all over, had a low-grade fever, and was exhausted. A raspy cough with a severe headache also plagued him, and for the first time that he could recall, he called the office and reported in sick. Karl treated himself with aspirin, which caused his fever to drop; however, the rest of his symptoms continued and he remained home in bed for the next five days. On the fifth day, he noticed that his urine was dark. *I'd better increase my fluids,* he reasoned, *I'm dehydrated from the fever.* He found that he could not remain awake beyond two in the afternoon and was not able to return to the job. After a few days more, Karl began to feel stronger and had completely forgotten that Sharon would be there the next evening. He had lost track of time during his illness, along with twelve pounds.

A knock on the door startled him for a moment. "Yes, who is it?" Karl said weakly.

"It's Sharon, Dad."

"Oh my goodness, I'm coming." He had been asleep since 2 p.m. He looked at his watch; it was already six, and he had totally forgotten Sharon was arriving to spend the weekend with him. He ambled to the door and opened it. His daughter was standing there with a small overnight bag slung over her shoulder. Karl sighed deeply. She looked just like her mother, and for a brief moment, it was as though he'd been transported thirty years back in time. He had been so much in love with her and had missed her immensely since her death over five years ago. In his own world, he imagined she was still alive and pictured vivid scenes of finding her again. He had even conjured up the exact details of their reunion, and it was this that kept him going. He relived the memories of his life with her as a defense against loneliness. Sometimes, he would pull out the photos and dwell over each one, trying to recall the events surrounding the picture. Only then would Karl relax with a drink and savor the memories. His life with Jenny had been beautiful, and the sorrow her death had left him with was devastating.

His eyes were now transfixed on Sharon's, who was also experiencing deep thought, but hers were of a different ilk. She was shocked at her dad's appearance. Standing there in the dimly lit doorway, he looked haggard and sickly. Quickly, she hugged him and kissed his face affectionately. Tears welled up in her eyes and she felt a lump in her throat. For a long moment, she couldn't speak. Karl told her he loved her and that she was beautiful just like her mother. This served to further the release of emotions in both of them, and they hugged and cried.

She squeezed him again around the waist, and Karl groaned and stiffened his body. "What's the matter, Dad? she asked. "Do you have pain?"

"My right side was painful for a second."

"That happened right when I hugged you. Let's go inside. I want to examine you."

They entered the condo and Sharon threw her bag in the guest bedroom. Karl proceeded to the kitchen to fix a pot of coffee. He called to Sharon to join him in the kitchen. She walked into the well-lit room and surveyed her father, then sat across the table from him. "Dad, you've lost weight. Haven't you been eating right?"

"Well, to tell you the truth, I've been sick for a week," he answered, nodding his head.

Sharon looked closer at his face and then got up and went over to him. She put her finger on his lower right eye lid and asked him to look up while she gently pulled the lower lid down.

"Dad, you are jaundiced! How long have you been like this?" she asked in exasperation.

"I didn't even notice, honestly," he confessed with total innocence.

Sharon was now worried, and her quick mind ran through the most likely possibilities. "What are your symptoms?" "I thought I had the flu. You know, fever, chills, muscle pain, lethargy and malaise," he rattled off to her.

"Did you have any abdominal pain?" she fired back.

"No, not really. If you're looking for a history of fatty food intolerance or right upper quadrant pain of gall bladder disease, you've struck out," he chided. How he loved to spar with her about medical issues. Karl was trying to minimize her concern over his illness, but it wasn't working very well. One look at her and he was well aware that her analytical mind was now in high gear.

"Have you noticed that your urine appeared very dark lately?"

"I haven't really paid attention to that … but I noticed it was darker than usual."

"What about the color of your stool?" She was trying to find out if there were signs of obstructive jaundice, which would be cause for extreme concern. That type of jaundice without pain was a big red flag for cancer of the pancreas. The organ sat in an anatomical position that caused obstructive jaundice by virtue of mechanical compression, and an enlarging tumor would occlude the bile duct at the point of its emptying into the duodenum. She knew the ominous outcome of pancreatic cancer and became very anxious as she thought about it.

"My stools have appeared normal."

She was relieved to hear his answer. "Dad, come into the den and lie down on the couch so I can examine your abdomen."

Karl obliged and lay on the couch while she felt his abdomen.

"Your liver is enlarged about six centimeters," she told him without any passion in her voice. "I think you need to have a panel of liver function tests done right away."

"Look, I feel much better now. It can wait until Monday." Sharon weighed the response in the light of her own anxiety which was driving her. "Okay, but I want your promise that you will have the tests Monday and fax me the results. I don't trust you to take care of yourself at all," she told him, laughing, and hugged him again.

"I promise. Now let's talk for a while." Karl admitted that his appetite had declined and he had lost twelve pounds in two weeks, but it was now improving and he felt stronger. Sharon told him she thought he might have hepatitis. After they debated all the health issues, she made dinner for both of them and they chatted about everything as well as nothing for the rest of the evening.

– 19 –

HEPATITIS PANDEMIC HITS THE U.S.

Sharon returned from her weekend visit with her father and was immediately caught up in a whirlwind of medical practice. The news media was hard at work documenting the latest public health reports on the tracking of the hepatitis virus. As expected, the CDC in Atlanta had confirmed that the virus had mutated again, enhancing its virulency. This caused patients to develop hepatic failure much more rapidly, thereby increasing the mortality rate. Those who were more fortunate received liver transplants.

World Health Care had arranged for the evaluation of twelve new patients for transplants. They were from the Southwest United States, and at the onset of their disease, the primary care doctors had drawn blood for genetic testing, unknown to the patients. Whenever the diagnosis of hepatitis was made by laboratory testing, the labs were instructed to forward blood samples to the research laboratory in Malibu for *further testing*. The lab was doing research in virology and required infected blood—or so went the propaganda promoted through the pipeline. In this manner, the lab could begin the genetic liver growth early in the disease process so that organs would be ready when needed for those afflicted with the dreaded illness. World Health Care realized very well they had an obligation to provide the liver transplants if medically necessary, and since they were fortunate to have joint ventured with Genome and Bently, the costs to them were nominal. The great majority of the American patients were children, just as it was in Europe.

Sharon had worked all day Monday and most of Tuesday evaluating the referred patients. She'd admitted half of them to the hospital in accordance with the predicted time of need so as to have the organ ready for transplant within a few days of the date of surgery. The remaining patients were put on the waiting Clone Garden List. These patients could wait for a few months before their transplant was necessary but were scheduled to be followed in Sharon's outpatient clinic and also by the gastroenterologist. The twelve patients were scheduled for transplant surgery rather quickly due to their clinical status. The first transplant was scheduled for the next day, with the rest to follow at the rate of two transplants daily. This meant operating straight through the weekend. Sharon contacted the research lab herself to verify the readiness of the donor cloned livers for her acute patients. She was pleasantly surprised when Dr. Matson informed her that all the livers were ready for the recipients. He also said how pleased he was that the primary care doctors caring for these patients had done an excellent job in keeping him informed regularly of the clinical status. They had developed a computer model to simulate the diseased hepatitis liver, wherein they used the blood enzymes values and the bilirubin levels to predict the rate of liver destruction. All the doctors responsible for the care of the patients had seen to it that the lab received the weekly blood test results for their "research program." As a result, they were able to obtain updated weekly computer model predictions as to the time when transplant surgery would have to be performed. It was easy for them to adjust the rate of liver cell growth in conjunction with the rate of disease process within the patient. In this manner, they not only produced the desired organ, but did so on time. They were now working on a similar program to predict the exact time of organ failure of hearts and lungs with the use of laboratory biochemical blood analysis. Here also, the cloned organ would be available when the recipient needed the transplant, thereby avoiding the risk of waiting.

That afternoon, Sharon received a call from her father while she was in her clinic. She hastened to her small office and closed the door.

"Hi Dad, how are you feeling?" she asked as though she hadn't seen him in months, when in reality she had only been gone two days.

"I feel better. I have the lab results for you, and I don't think you'll like them," he said somberly.

Sharon felt the panic cut her to the quick and bit her lower lip. After she regained her composure, she asked, "What are they, Dad?" She scavenged her desk for something to write on and found her pen quickly.

"The SGOT is 850, the SGPT is 1200, and the GGT is

1050. The bilirubin is 6.4 total and the rest of the tests are all normal."

"You have hepatitis, Dad, I'm seventy-five percent sure of it. Will you call the lab and ask them to run a hepatitis profile? If they need more blood, please go back right away."

"I knew you'd say that, so I beat you to the punch. They will have the results in two days. In the meantime, I will stay at home. I don't want to infect anyone with this virus."

"That's great. Get some rest."

"The newspapers say you are feeling the brunt of the hepatitis epidemic down there."

"Yes, the epidemic has hit us very hard. We're doing a lot of transplants on kids."

"That reminds me, is there a test for the new virus?" asked Karl.

"I don't know. That's a good question. I didn't even give it a second thought, but there may not be because it's such a novelty. I'll find out and let you know. Call me with the results when you get them back on Thursday. Gotta run, love you Dad," she said with tenderness.

"See you later. Love you too, Sharon."

Sharon placed a call to Dr. Matson at the Research Lab and waited while they tracked his whereabouts and finally connected her.

"Dr. Matson, this is Sharon Dell at TWMC. How are you today?"

"Very well, thank you Dr. Dell. How may I help you?"

"Tell me, have you identified the epidemic hepatitis antigen yet?"

"Yes, we have. We have named it the hepatitis D2 virus. It is a direct mutant of the hepatitis D virus. We have it well typed and identified."

"Do you have a commercial lab test available to detect its presence?"

"As a matter of fact we do, and we are also in commercial production for the vaccine."

"That's wonderful. When will the vaccine be available for worldwide immunization usage?"

"The first batch will be ready next week. We will only have a limited amount, so we want to immunize all hospital personnel at TWMC first, and when the rest is available in a month, we will supply the health departments within the U.S. They placed their orders when we notified them a few months ago of our progress in this area."

"Great! I have a special favor to ask you now. My dad may have hepatitis. I don't know whether it is hepatitis D2 or not. Would you test his blood for me if I send you a sample?"

"I would be happy to. When will you send it?"

"I am going to call the lab and request they forward you a sample today if possible. Certainly by Thursday at the latest."

"Fine, I'll look for it and will call you back as soon as I have the results."

"Thank you so much, Dr. Matson. I'll await your call."

"Goodbye, Dr. Dell." She returned to her patients and began to write her evaluation in each chart.

The next day, she made a special effort to arrive at the cafeteria earlier in hopes of seeing Michael. She looked around and saw him sitting alone at the same lunch table they had occupied a few weeks before. Michael looked up and caught her eye, motioning her to join him. As she approached, he rose and pulled the chair from the table for her.

Sharon felt slightly flushed as she took the chair, as though everyone in the room were watching her. She looked around and didn't see anyone staring and felt relieved. Michael broke the silence. "Have you been on a hunger strike? I haven't seen you here in almost two weeks."

"I've had to eat at odd times because of my schedule and my father's illness."

"What's the matter with your dad?"

"He has hepatitis and I'm really concerned."

"Why?"

"Well, the enzymes are high and he just looks horrible. I'm waiting for the results of further tests."

"I am so sorry," he said with compassion. "I hope he improves soon."

"Thank you." She felt better now that she had someone to talk to about her concerns, and smiled. "What have you been doing lately?"

"I'm putting the final touch on a paper I'm submitting for publication."

"Really? What is it about?"

"It's a research project concerning the role of genes in breast cancer."

"That's great. I know there are exciting breakthroughs in the area."

"Say if you aren't busy one evening," said Michael with a grin, "why don't you let me tell you more about it over dinner?"

"That would be great," she responded, so quickly that she surprised herself. "I have to run. Give me a call."

– 20 –

THE LEARNING MODE

The liver transplants had been going very well without complications until Thursday evening, when Henry Diaz was admitted for an acute rejection process. Sharon had done his liver transplant four months ago and he had been doing well on all his visits to the clinic. As noted by Barry Swenz, all the liver function tests were normal. Henry was only five years old and had contracted the dreaded hepatitis D2 virus and then undergone a successful transplant operation. His mother brought him into the emergency room with a history of vomiting and abdominal pain that had been occurring off and on for two weeks. She had noticed that his urine was dark and his stool the day before had appeared clay-colored. As if that weren't enough, he also had a temperature of 103 degrees. The child was evaluated by Dr. Shore, who was the intern rotating through the emergency room for the month.

"Let's get external cooling measures on this kid, stat!" he barked at Janet, the ER nurse. "Also, pull a CBC and liver panel." Janet Crosby had been around ERs for ages, and what she had forgotten about the treatment of patients in crisis, the good Dr. Paul Shore would probably never know. She had seen the inexperienced interns come and go, and was more of a gruff, understanding mother to them than a nurse. She guided her young wards toward the proper treatment of emergencies and, in most cases, had already done what was indicated before any intern had even organized his treatment plan. Janet had taken the history from Mrs. Diaz and had already begun the cooling measures a good ten minutes before his excellency, Dr. Shore, ever examined the patient. In addition, she'd also inserted a 325-grain Tylenol suppository into the boy in order to reduce the fever before it caused seizures to occur.

Shore examined Henry's abdomen and auscultated his chest. Neurologically, he seemed normal, but periodically, he was shaking violently all over. "Let's get a CAT scan of his head," he shouted. "I want to rule out a CNS problem!" Shore was very impressed with himself and wanted those within hearing range of his voice to be cognizant of his genius also. Janet rolled her eyes upward and exhaled against slightly pursed lips. The ER was swamped, and there were at least thirty more patients in the waiting room still waiting to be seen. She knew that to order a CT scan would tie up the ER for an additional two hours, and this was just unacceptable.

Janet wielded immense power at TWMC due to her twenty-five years of dedication and her nursing excellence. She had been the ER supervisor for years, and through her single-handed efforts, molded it into the most enviable emergency department in the Southern California area. The efficiency of operation, as well as the quality of care administered, had achieved accolades from all of the licensing and examining bureaucrats in the state. It was this fact that empowered her. When she wanted something done, all she had to do was request it, and James Foxworthy stumbled over himself to do her bidding. He, of course, also received praises from everyone which, in reality, were all a result of Janet's keen and dedicated mind. She was a rare individual who believed that the Peter Principle was very real. Even though she had obtained a Ph.D. in Nursing Administration, she would not leave the clinical field for any sum of money. Janet knew that in order to be a good administrator, one had to keep their hand in the clinical aspects of nursing. If one drifted too far from the new advances of the profession, one's knowledge became obsolete, which directly affected the ability to properly administrate a department.

She walked over to Dr. Shore and asked to speak with him immediately.

"I am too busy to talk right now," he retorted in annoyance.

"Dr. Shore, this is important and will only take five minutes." She led him out of the chaos of the ER and into the small doctor's office at the end of the hallway. He followed her reluctantly and sat in the chair behind the small desk as she closed the door.

"Well, what is it?"

"Henry Diaz does not have a CNS problem in my estimation," she said softly, so as not to be threatening to the young doctor. Shore had already heard via the grapevine of Janet's prowess and power. Furthermore, it had been rumored that her personal assessment of each doctor rotating through the ER was paramount in what the ER physician director decided to write in his evaluation. But his pompous ego won out and he barked at her, "What are you talking about? You are not the doctor here, I am, and I call the shots!"

"Perhaps you could enlighten me then as to what central nervous system illness you are attempting to diagnose?" she answered politely. She had been through this before and was well seasoned in her abilities to withstand strong egos.

Shore saw this as a threat rather than an opportunity to perhaps teach this nurse something. "This child might have a subdural hematoma from trauma or a brain abscess," he snorted with a quick, haughty turn of his head.

"Doctor Shore, why would you consider a subdural when there is no history of trauma?"

Shore thought for a moment and found that he really didn't have a plausible answer to the question.

Sensing his embarrassment and wanting to deflate the issue to avoid hostility, she continued, "Also, Doctor, why a brain abscess?"

"He had a violent grand mal seizure twice while I was examining him. You were there, didn't you see it?" he asked calmly.

"I think, although I could be in error, Henry was having rigors, not seizures," she suggested without emotion.

Shore was stopped dead in his tracks in his thought processes. *Could I have mistaken a shaking chill for a seizure?* He saw a chance to resurrect his falling ego. "What would be the cause of such a chill? He has liver rejection that will be confirmed by the lab tests, I'll bet!"

"Well, for openers, a brain abscess would have had to be

caused by an infection that was ongoing for a while. There is no such history here. In fact, the child had only been ill for a few days. I think that would effectively eliminate a brain abscess as a real possibility. What it sounds like to me is that he has a possible obstruction of the common bile duct. He acts like an adult with a biliary tract obstruction or an acute gall bladder."

"If that is so, what is causing the rigors?" he asked smugly. He had already conceded his position in his own mind because this made good sense to him. He knew the only reason he'd ordered a CT of the head was for the sake of completion. "When you don't know, test by the shotgun method. Maybe something will find a target!"

"I have seen this before, Doctor. I really would consider, if I were you, the possibility of septicemia from biliary obstruction."

It rang true and found its mark. He sat down and shook his head. "You know, you may be right. Let's get blood cultures and cancel the CT Scan." He felt relieved when he saw her smile. "Certainly, Doctor! You know what, it takes a very special person to admit they may have made an error. You are very special in my book." She walked over to him and put her arms around his waist and gave him a big hug. He hugged her back, and suddenly all the threat melted away. Shore felt confident.

"You're also a wonderful person, as well as the smartest nurse I've met."

"Remember in the future, Doctor, nurses care for the patients twenty-four hours a day, while the doctor only sees the patient for, at most, twenty minutes during that time frame. You can glean a lot more about your patient if you read the nurses' notes and discuss the patient with the nurse." She wanted to make certain that he would always remember to confide in the nurses and listen to their suggestions for the care of each patient.

They heard a rapping on the door. "Yes, come in," said Shore.

The door opened and an ER technician handed the lab reports to Dr. Shore. He glanced at them and turned to Janet. "The enzymes are high normal, which is against rejection, and the bilirubin is 7.1 with the direct at 6. You're right, this is an obstructive jaundice. Let's get a CT of the bile ducts and call Dr. Dell to fill her in."

Janet smiled and thought, *He'll be a good one, because he can listen.*

Sharon Dell arrived at the ER within an hour and discussed the case with Shore. To his credit, he told her the entire story, including the fact that he had initially barked up the wrong tree, but after receiving help from Janet been able to correctly diagnose the problem. Janet interrupted him to tell Sharon that all the credit should go to Shore. Shore blushed while the two women smiled.

Sharon saw the CT Scan and pointed out that the common bile duct at the point just below its connection to the cystic duct was markedly constricted, whereas the duct proximal to it was ballooned, as well as both the hepatic ducts. There was no question that an obstruction had occurred at the point of suturing the donor's common bile duct to the native one. This had been the result of scar tissue developing since the transplant surgery. She complimented Dr. Shore on the fact that he had started Henry on appropriate intravenous antibiotic therapy, which no doubt was the most important factor in saving his life. Blood-borne bacteria from the biliary tract might well have caused the demise of the patient had antibiotics not been promptly administered.

Shore realized were it not for the timely intervention by Janet, he wouldn't have started antibiotics until the CT scan of the head had been obtained. That would have been at least two or more additional hours, and he might now have been lamenting an untoward outcome. He felt very good about himself and vowed to always keep an open mind in every clinical situation. In this case, the ordering of an inappropriate procedure would have delayed the proper treatment of the patient and could have easily caused a fatality. Henry was taken to the radiology department, where Sharon watched while the gastroenterologist performed an endoscopy procedure on the anesthetized patient. The scope was passed into Henry's stomach then into the first portions of the duodenum. The ampulla of Vater was identified and the duct cannulated with the fiberoptic scope. It was determined that the duct was free from stones and the constriction was the result of scar tissue. The suturing together of the genetic donor's duct to the patient's had resulted in heavy scarring, which markedly narrowed the lumen of the bile duct, thus allowing bacteria to grow abundantly in the sludge. A balloon was inserted and advanced to the point of narrowing. Once the balloon was in place, it was inflated and the constricted area dilated.

The entire procedure took about two-and-a-half hours from start to finish. Sharon spoke with the resident who would be directly responsible for Henry's care and alerted him that she wanted to be called for any problems. She went home to shower and dress before returning to the hospital for her routine. She was exhausted, but it didn't matter to her. This was her whole life, and she loved every minute of it.

-21-

ALL THAT GLITTERS IS NOT GOLD

The next few days saw the bilirubin dropping and Henry acting normal, since his fever had not raised its ugly head in almost thirty-six hours. During this time, his bilirubin level dropped, the fever defervesced, and his conditioned improved. Then, with no warning, Henry spiked to 104 degrees with shaking chills and severe abdominal pain. The floor nurses called the resident physician, who quickly notified Sharon as she had requested. She came to the child's room immediately and was met by Dr. Ted Evans, the resident.

"What were your findings on examination, Dr. Evans?" asked Sharon.

"His lungs are clear and the heart is normal. There is no costo-vertebral tenderness, which rules out the kidney as a cause, but he has extreme guarding and rebound tenderness of the abdomen."

"That doesn't sound good. Let's check him again." They both went to the bedside. Sharon pulled the sheets down and placed her hands on the abdomen only after she had warmed them up by rubbing them together. Although very lethargic, Henry screamed when she palpated his abdomen. Palpation of all four quadrants of the abdomen resulted in a similar response. When she gently exerted firm pressure then abruptly withdrew her hand, Henry screamed again. "Okay Dr. Evans, what is the diagnosis?" she asked.

"It's obviously a case of peritonitis."

"What is the cause?"

"Well, it could be a ruptured appendix or even a ruptured Meckles diverticulum."

"Sure it might, but why reach for a diagnosis when there is one that is in reach?"

"I don't follow you."

"What is the most important aspect of a patient evaluation?"

"You mean the physical exam?"

"No, I mean the history. Always remember, you will be able to make the diagnosis on the majority of your patients by the history."

"Even so, the history was unobtainable because of the age of the patient."

"Certainly, I agree. However, you do have the patient's chart—a wonderful record of what Henry has had done since his admission here!"

"I am familiar with his case. He had a balloon dilatation of the common bile duct performed a few days ago."

"Exactly! What are the possible complications of that procedure.?"

"Oh no. He's got bile peritonitis! The duct was ruptured by the balloon inadvertently."

"That's correct. What is the treatment for it?"

"Surgery to repair the duct and insertion of a tube to drain the bile proximal to the tear in the duct. Oh yes, and also, I would start antibiotics immediately."

"Good job, Doctor. Remember, always review the history thoroughly. Get Henry ready for surgery. I'll meet you in the OR in one hour."

– 22 –

THE LABEL
TELLS IT ALL

D r. Matson had received the blood sample from Karl
Dell, and the testing confirmed the diagnosis of hepatitis D2. The enzymes revealed he had a fulminant infection,
and the computer anticipated the need for a liver transplant
in four weeks. He discussed this with Dr. Cook.

"How could his liver be so far gone in such a short time?
The history is that he became ill two weeks ago, and yet the
degree of liver necrosis appears as though he's been infected
for at least six weeks," said Matson.

"The only answer is that he must have received a massive
inoculum somehow."

"The computer says it would be impossible to have acquired that amount of virus by the usual body entry methods," said Matson.

"That leaves only one route then. He had to have been
inoculated directly with the virus."

"How could that be? We are the only ones who have the virus growing in culture."

"I don't have the slightest. I'm going to the lab to see if they have identified any radio nuclear tags on the virus we recovered from his blood sample. It will only take me five minutes to go there and find the results."

"I think we should notify Mike Rome and David Malkin about this," said Cook sternly. He dialed the extension to Mike Rome's office. "Bring back the results, Victor—I'll be speaking with Rome."

The man answered quickly. "How is the research coming, Dr. Cook?" asked Rome.

"The research is right on schedule, sir. We are producing the immune hepatitis vaccine in large quantities and we have corrected the deficiency in the KZ67. It won't be necessary to continue its use after twenty-four months in transplant patients."

"How did the blood test turn out on Sharon's father? I know you told me the other day you were awaiting his sample."

"He has the most severe case of hepatitis we have seen to date, and we know he had to have been injected with the live virus. The computer has calculated the dose he must have received in order to be this sick, and it couldn't have been acquired in the standard manner of infectivity."

"Maybe he stuck himself with an infected needle," answered Rome flippantly.

"That's impossible. The load of virus couldn't be that much from a contaminated needle stick. We are the only ones who have the live virus cultures, and there is a vial of cultured virus missing from our lab. Dr. Matson just handed me the inventory that he completed. Someone has used our virus to inject into Dr. Karl Dell!"

"How can you be so certain?" asked Rome with some hesitancy and the slightest bit of tremor in his voice.

Matson entered the room in excitement and handed a written report to Cook. Cook read it and quickly resumed his phone conversation.

"We tag our virus with a radio nuclear identification. It's an isotope label we attached. We have identified that specific label in the virus recovered from Dr. Dell's blood."

There was a strained silence. "Do you anticipate the need for a liver transplant for Karl Dell?"

"The computer projects the need for a transplant in three to four weeks." "Well then," replied Rome, "it seems to me that we should start the genetic cloning program for a new liver immediately. Can we grow one for Sharon's dad in time?" he asked with uncertainty.

"We can now clone a liver faster by using the patient's liver cells directly. If we can get a liver biopsy performed quickly, I'm sure that we can clone the cell immediately. We have refined the method to enhance and enlarge cell growth with liver cells, so I believe we can have a liver ready in three to four weeks rather than using bone marrow and waiting four to six weeks," replied Cook with pride. "We'll have to wait until she calls us for help first, though. We are not supposed to know anything at this point—wait a minute, why can't we tell her that we routine run a computer model on hepatitis bloods and the diagnosis of hepatitis is uncertain? A tissue diagnosis is necessary. I'm certain she will be amenable to a liver biopsy. I'll call her myself."

"Great, then we will be able to offer Sharon some valuable help for her father. Let me know how it's going."

"We still have the question of who had access to the virus, and moreover who would have done such a thing," said Cook.

"I don't know, but we definitely have a security problem. I will discuss this with Dave Malkin, but in the meanwhile, I want you to meet with Dr. Peter Harper. We have just assigned him to work with you in the Research Lab. I will refer your concern to the security chief, who will investigate it for us.

"Dr. Harper is with New Jersey Medical School. Do you know of his research?" asked Cook innocently.

"If you mean the research he has published concerning the method by which a cell is programmed to live or die, then yes," answered Rome in a very snotty manner.

"I'm sorry, but since this is hot-off-the-press research, I didn't think you would know of it. The process is called *apoptosis*," replied Cook apologetically.

"Whatever, he will be calling you. Allow him to set up his own research lab after he talks to you about it," ordered Rome.

"I certainly will. Goodbye," said Cook.

"Victor, did you hear that? Peter Harper will be joining us."

"That will sure be an enhancement to our program. When?" asked Victor eagerly.

"He's to call shortly, and we'll meet together to hear about his research plans."

"Call me whenever. I have to leave now."

"I'm returning to the lab myself."

-23-

THE OMINOUS MEETING

Karl Dell wasn't feeling well at all. He'd continued to lose weight and now felt weak most of the time. His skin was bruising easily, and large black-and-blue spots covered his arms. His face was drawn and his muscle mass had diminished in size, both as a result of disuse as well as his liver's failure to make protein. He called Southwest Airlines and booked a seat on the 5 p.m. flight to Ontario, then called Sharon.

"Sharon, I am getting worse. I'm worried!" said Karl in a low voice.

"What's the matter with your voice, Dad?" she asked with alarm.

"I'm just so weak I can't speak any louder."

"Are you able to fly down here, or shall I drive up to pick you up?"

"I can get to the airport."

"I want you to fly down here right away. I think you may need to be in the hospital. I'll admit you here at TWMC."

She would tell him about the necessary liver biopsy, which she'd just been informed about by Doctor Cook. There was no sense in alarming Karl now about the possibility that he might have something other than hepatitis affecting his liver.

"I won't argue with you. I will fly down tonight. I have tickets on the five o'clock out of Sacramento and I'll take a shuttle to TWMC. I'll call your office when I arrive. See you then."

Sharon was shocked at the response. He had bought the flight tickets already; that was not like her dad. *He must really be feeling rotten.* She looked at her watch. It was shortly after one, and she had her clinic to attend.

At 7:50 p.m., Sharon was called by the hospital switchboard operator to notify her that her father was in the lobby. She ran out of her office and quickly entered the elevator that deposited her on the first floor. Walked to the front of the lobby, she found her father sitting in a chair. "Oh my God, Dad, why didn't you call me sooner?" Karl was gaunt and had dropped another ten pounds. The skin on his face was drawn so tight that the hollows of the eye sockets were dramatized. His arms were black and blue and his skin was golden yellow. Sharon called the ER and had them bring a wheelchair to the lobby. Karl was too weak to complain as she followed him to the ER, where she signed him in and called the on-call resident physician to admit him and perform a percutaneous liver biopsy immediately.

After he received fresh frozen plasma to correct the clotting factor deficiencies, the liver biopsy was performed and sent to the Research Lab by special courier. It was about four hours later when she finally discussed the case with Dr.

Mallis, the medical resident. He informed her of all his findings. Karl's liver was very small, indicating hepatic collapse
due to the loss of liver cells that had been destroyed by the
D2 virus. He was bleeding into the skin as well as the intestines because the liver was not making the necessary clotting
proteins. The liver function tests showed the bilirubin was
over 16 and the enzymes were in the 300 range.

This was an ominous sign, Sharon knew. The enzymes
should have been higher but since there wasn't much left of
the organ, there wasn't much remaining for the virus to kill.
The end result was a lower than expected enzyme marker of
a dying liver. He was also suffering the effects of the liver
failure on his brain. The liver was not removing ammonia
from the blood, and this was toxic to the central nervous system. All the necessary supportive therapy was initiated, but
Karl would need a liver, that was abundantly plain to Sharon.
The problem, however, was that Karl was not a World Health
Care HMO patient and, therefore, he would normally have to
await his turn on the waiting list. Generally, a patient had to
wait a minimum of four months for a donor liver to become
available. Sharon slumped in her chair and closed her eyes.
Abruptly, she came to life and seized her telephone.

"This is Dr. Dell, I must speak with Mr. Rome."

"I am sorry, but he has gone for the day and won't be back
until tomorrow," replied the telephone exchange operator.

"Don't you have a way to reach him?" cried Sharon.

"Oh no, we never call Mr. Rome at home. I can reach Dr.
Matson for you, though."

"Please do. Thank you." The exchange operator left the

line for a few minutes and then Sharon heard the familiar click as the phone lines were connected.

"Dr. Dell, what can I do for you?" asked Matson.

"Dr. Matson, my dad was just admitted with liver failure and he will need a liver transplant very soon. Is there any way I can get one for him?" She began to cry.

"I'm sure there is, Dr. Dell. I am certain you'll hear from Mr. Rome tomorrow. Get some rest, you sound exhausted."

"Thanks, I will." That night she found it difficult to sleep. Thoughts rolled about in her head as though they were in a clothes dryer.

Sharon visited her dad the next morning and noticed he was slightly confused. His ammonia levels were climbing because the liver was challenged by the process of incorporating huge amounts of ammonia into other products. The excessive ammonia was the product of all the extra bleeding within the intestines, which was being digested by bacteria, and in the process ammonia was released. Since the liver was so damaged, its capacity to filter the ammonia from the blood and change it into a nontoxic product was diminished. His abdomen was distended because of the development of ascites. The pathophysiology of ascites was well understood. When the liver failed to make sufficient amounts of albumin, resulting in a lowered osmotic pressure in the blood, it led to the outpouring of plasma into the free peritoneal space. The high portal venous pressure resulted in altered mechanics of fluid exchange across the peritoneal membrane, and the plasma leaked into the abdominal cavity. She knew his liver was at the end of its usefulness and convinced Karl to sign a consent for the liver transplant.

Her pager sounded and she read the message. Mike Rome was calling her. Picking up the nurse's phone, she called the operator and told her to forward the call to her office. She left the floor hurriedly to get there.

Coming through the door to her secretary's office, she told her to put the call through on her phone and hold all others. Sharon ran into her office, closed the door as she entered, and grabbed at the ringing telephone. She slumped her weary body into the chair.

"Hello, Mr. Rome. Thank you for calling."

"Good morning, Sharon. How is your father doing today?" he asked.

"He's stable but slowly losing ground. I believe he will need a new liver within the week."

"That's what I wanted to speak with you about. Can we meet for lunch today?"

"I am extremely busy today, but perhaps we can meet this evening."

"That would be fine. Mr. Malkin will be with me also. How about Spago on Sunset Blvd? At eight?"

"I'm sure I can be there by eight." "We'll look forward to it. See you then."

He hung the phone up and buzzed his secretary. "Please call Spago and arrange reservations for dinner tonight at eight for four. When you're done, call David Malkin and Dr. Peter Harper to meet me here at seven and we'll all go in my car."

Sharon thought it was a nice gesture for Michael Rome

to ask her to dinner at the fashionable Spago. She had always heard such good reports about the food, but was always too busy to try it out. *I wonder what he wants to talk about?*

The rest of the day was crammed with decision-making issues. Surgeries were planned and patients examined. She had to attend a faculty meeting at noon, which was among the less important things to do. In between activities, Sharon checked on her father's progress. The liver functions showed a marked reduction in the enzymes, which on first glance, appeared to be a sign of improvement. However, this was in conjunction with a rising bilirubin, and it indicated that the liver was failing miserably. The reason for the drastic fall in the enzyme values, she again surmised, was that there was not much normal tissue left for the virus to destroy, as was confirmed by the resident's examination—the liver was shrinking. This was all extremely ominous. She hoped the genetic liver would be available soon.

At 5 p.m., Sharon left for home, where she quickly bathed and dressed. She was on the 10 Freeway westbound by 6:15 and pulled up to Spago at 7:30, where a valet dressed in a red vest took her car as he handed her a yellow ticket. Sharon entered the spacious foyer of the restaurant. Quickly, she spotted the rest room and entered it. She checked her appearance and then walked back into the grandiose waiting area. In the center was situated the most spectacular display of flowers she had ever seen. The huge vase was overflowing with white and purple orchids complemented by various bright orange and blue blossoms intertwined with the yellows and whites. She gaped at the arrangement and couldn't believe they were real, so she cautiously extended her hand and felt the petals. They were! She walked to the restaurant's door and announced herself to the maitre d', who escorted her to her awaiting dinner companions.

As she approached the spacious table, she was met by three gentlemen, all of whom stood up when she approached. She realized she was the center of attention as she noticed heads turning from the nearby tables, giving witness to her beauty. *Maybe I should frequent this place again,* she thought as she scanned the men's faces following after her. Sharon had always been too busy with her professional life to take advantage of any social relationships and therefore had missed out on dining in places like Spago. She was entranced by it all.

"I see you found it okay," said Rome. "You remember David Malkin, CEO of Bently Drug Corporation, and may I present Dr. Peter Halper. Dr. Halper has joined our research team."

"Your reputation precedes you, Dr. Dell," said Halper.

"I hope your father is comfortable," said Malkin.

"He is very ill but seems to be holding his own."

"Why don't we all order drinks and relax a bit. It's been a devil of a day," said Rome with a smile. He signaled the attentive waiter, who arrived in a flurry and took the drink orders.

Sharon ordered her favorite, a Vermouth Cassis, which she nursed for thirty minutes while their small talk covered the local news events of the day, as well as sports, of course. Finally, they ordered dinner, which wasn't nearly soon enough for Sharon, who hadn't eaten since noon. The conversation eventually came around to the reason for their meeting. "Dr.

Dell, we have asked you to join us so we might discuss a few issues relative to your father's health problem," began Rome.

"What do you wish to discuss?" replied Sharon with concern.

"Please don't take offense, but we are disturbed over the fact that your father audited TWMC for the DOC a month ago or so," said Rome.

"I don't understand your concern."

"Please let me continue," he stated, paying no attention to her reply. "We all felt a sense of betrayal. We thought we had your assurance that our research was safe with you, but when your father appeared on the scene, I must confess, I believed you had informed him of our secret."

"That is preposterous! I have never said a thing to my father about the research," she replied in indignation. Her eyes were ablaze as she stared into Rome's with fury.

"Please Dr. Dell, I am only being truthful about our concerns, but I'm delighted to hear you say that. You know how much is at stake here, both in time and money, not to mention the lives that are now and will continue to be saved. We have to safeguard our projects and our stockholders."

"Just what are you getting at?" Sharon was angry at the insinuation she had "blown the whistle."

"You are aware, I'm sure, that we have no obligation to provide your father a cloned liver for transplant; however, we want to do it for him, and for you as well. All we require from you is your word you will not reveal any of our secrets. More specifically, we want your word that you won't testify against us in any legal proceeding."

Sharon cringed at the words. Why would this even be brought up?

"I am going to allow David to continue at this point."

David Malkin placed his drink on the table. "Here is where we stand. You possess very confidential information which may prove to be catastrophic if it were used against us in any manner, but especially in a court proceeding. We have therefore devised a way for us to be insured that you will never reveal anything. I am sorry if you are taken aback, but this is business ... and I mean big business. In order for you to understand better, we have asked Dr. Halper to present the process he developed. I assume you will accept our offer to supply the cloned liver for your father?"

"Of course I will."

The entrée was served and the conversation temporarily was suspended. Although it was impeccable in preparation and presentation, Sharon lost her appetite.

"In that case, I'll ask Dr. Halper to continue," he said with a smirk. Halper finished his drink. "My area of research has been in the field of cell injury and death. We have discovered what makes a cell live and die. All cells of the body, with the exception of those in the central nervous system, repair as well as regenerate new cells. We call the distinct form of cellular death wherein the cell actively participates in its own death apoptosis. We have discovered the regulation of cell death or survival is the result of certain genes. In this case, the gene is Bcl-2 and Bax, and their protein production will program the outcome. When the Bcl-2 protein is in excess, the cell will live, but when Bax is in excess, the cell will die.

This is what regulates the process of aging and is responsible for all of our organs growing new cells throughout life.

"We have developed a method to signal the cell to induce cellular death by increasing the production of Bax protein. We use the global positioning system to accomplish this feat; however, we have modified it slightly. As you may know, the GPS is a receiving unit equipped with the technology to receive radio signals in the Gigahertz frequency range. These are the signals sent continuously by hovering satellites, and the GPS frequency receiver then calculates where the receiver is located by interpreting the reception of these signals. We have devised technology that allows us to receive the same signal sent to the GPS chip residing in the liver. Then we are able to send a similar Gigahertz frequency radio code directly by our computer to the microchip that is located in the donor organ. The code is identified by the chip, and the chip emits electromagnetic energy that causes genetic disruption, which results in an overabundance of the Bax protein that is coded for by the Bax genes."

"Oh my God, are you telling me that the donor liver has an imbedded microchip in it and you expect me to insert that liver into my father?"

"The way we see it, you don't have a viable option, Dr. Dell—not if you are to save your father's life!" replied Rome, his tone sarcastic.

Sharon was livid. To implant a liver in her father that had a time bomb ready to detonate was more than she could bear. "You are all despicable human beings! I have never violated my pledge to secrecy. I thought you were all responsible members of society bent on a dedicated mission for the world. But I was misled. You are all in it just for the money! You are all cold-blooded, diabolic people ... scum of the world!"

"Dr. Dell," interrupted Malkin, "you are being extremely unfair. Our company has spent millions of dollars in the research and development phase in order to get to this point in time. We are about to recapture our investment and perhaps make profits. We are a public company and we have a fiduciary responsible to our investors to make profits. Contrary to what you think, profit is not something to be ashamed of—rather, it is the very essence of a free society. Insurance is also part and parcel of living in the U.S. We have to have our products insured. Look at it as a liability insurance for us. If the necessity for activating the policy never presents itself, then we shall never use it." He looked directly into Sharon's eyes and saw that she was full of hate and anger. She answered him not aloud but within her own mind, knowing well that she needed the liver, and fast. There was nothing to be gained in further discussion. "I said before and I say again now, your secret is safe. I shall not divulge it to anyone." Sharon thought about the description of the way in which the chip was programmed to deliver a sustained electromagnetic force so as to induce cellular death through the process of apoptosis. She had been informed also that this was the process that was increasingly being recognized as the key in normal development physiology as well as the development of cancer. The electromagnetic field disturbance acted by interfering in the cell division phase when all chromosomes duplicated, passing on its genetic complement to the newly formed cell. If the alignment of the chromosomes was altered at the mitosis or normal cell division process stage, the genes became modified and mutated, with the end result in the coding process to increase the production of Bax protein that turned the cellular signal on for cell death. The cell, once containing the abnormal gene, continued to pass its mutants to all further cells derived through the normal process of cell mitosis.

She thought about it for a few minutes and said nothing. It was hard for her to believe the entire scenario. The global positioning system that was so readily available as a precise navigational tool had now become the Sword of Damocles that would hang forever over her father's head. It amazed her how simplistic and yet how complex it all was, but more than that, it could be explained in only a few minutes. Years of research and tons of money came down to a two-minute explanation and a few moments of recall. She mellowed at the thought that, after the operation, her father would become normal again. After dwelling on this for a moment, she looked at Rome. "When will the liver be available?"

"Dr. Matson said it is now ready. We can have it to TWMC tomorrow if you wish to schedule surgery then," replied Rome with renewed invigoration. His bonuses were tied to the profitability of the company, as were David Malkin's, and both companies stood to do very well with the release of the hepatitis antigen and the new KZ67 anti-rejection drug. These were going to be distributed worldwide, not to mention the profits there would be from the sale of genetic organs to the world's transplant market as soon as the FDA approved them for public consumption. The European market already had a head start and there were glowing reports of success from those doing the clinical research.

"I will schedule surgery for tomorrow at ten a.m., then. I should leave now—I've got a long drive home."

"Thank you for coming, Dr. Dell. I am certain we will all be happier after your father's surgery. Please accept all of our wishes for a successful operation tomorrow."

~24~

TREATING YOUR OWN

B arry Swenz was aggravated. When he'd heard Sharon's dad had performed the medical chart audit at TWMC, he'd become enraged with Sharon. There was no question in his mind she was attempting to torpedo him, along with the research program. He had worked very hard to provide the best medical care available to the transplant patients, notwithstanding his own surgical skills in restoring lost extremities to accident victims. Besides that, he was going to receive enough money from the company to retire, if he wanted to. All his dreams that stemmed from the money were shattered by Sharon. He could not take the chance she might testify against him or the companies. It was just too much risk for him to bear. He called a colleague friend to ask questions about the development of certain research that had been mentioned in the meeting with Sharon.

The package was delivered to Barry at his hospital office by a messenger. He removed the parcel from the Igloo and placed it safely in his pocket. The messenger left the hospital with icebox in hand while Barry went into his office and looked at the vial of clear liquid. The label said *hepatitis D2 Antigen, made by Research Laboratories.* He placed a call to Sharon's office and was told she was in surgery and was not expected until 7 p.m. This agitated him further. He'd try again later.

In surgery, Sharon operated on her father with the objectivity that only could be summoned by a superwoman. Indeed, she was every bit of that, as she continued the tedious procedure of removing the small, collapsed liver and started the surgery for attachment of the donor liver to the bile ducts and blood vessels. She would not allow herself the luxury of a moment's rest during the procedure, because she could not let herself think about her patient. He was her flesh and blood lying under her scalpel. He needed to be a neutral body that required her touch of life, not her beloved father. That was the only way she could visualize her situation. She was almost ready to remove the diseased organ, and asked the circulating nurse to bring the donor liver closer so she might take a quick glance at it. *It's amazing,* she thought. *The liver is the perfect size and it has been engineered as such in the lab from the start.* She began the tedious task before her. Her thoughts were again of her father's illness. *How were they able to grow the liver to size so fast?* It had only been a few weeks since she'd had that phone call from Dr. Cook. In order for a liver to grow to the adult required size, it had to have been started a good month at least before he called her. That meant they had to have begun the cloning process four to five weeks before the call. *But how could they have possibly accomplished it?* They had to have had her father's bone marrow to do it. *Oh no! They knew he would need a liver, and that means they had to do computer modeling to evaluate the length of time it would take for the virus to destroy the organ. This would give them a date to shoot for. Why would they even consider computer evaluation for the need of a transplant? Dad wasn't that sick then, and he had only been ill for a few weeks at the most. They had to suspect that he would require a liver and wanted to have one ready for him, but they never told me that when the test results were reported to me. They led me to believe a liver biopsy was needed to confirm the diagnosis. Now why would they expect him to become so ill as to need a transplant?*

There was only one answer. They must have known he acquired a massive load of virus. But how could they possibly have know that? The thoughts continued to revolve in her head without resolution.

The operation had gone without a problem. Upon its completion, all vital signs were stable, and it was now up to the new organ to cleanse the blood of toxins and to get rid of the bilirubin. She breathed deeply and walked to the doctors' lounge for a moment of relaxation before she dictated the operative report. Returning to her office, she saw that there was a note that Barry had called her. She dialed his office and waited for him to pick up the phone.

"Hi Sharon, do you have a moment to talk?" he asked.

"Sure."

"First things first. How did your Dad's surgery go today?" he asked earnestly.

"It went very well, thank you for asking. I think he will do just fine."

"Glad to hear it. Dr. Matson sent over a batch of hepatitis D2 vaccine for us to immunize ourselves. May I bring a vial over for you?"

"Yes, that would be very nice of you. We should all be immunized."

"I'll be right over then."

He hung up the phone and smiled. Ten minutes later, he walked into Sharon's office with the vial. "Well, I'm here to help stamp out disease," he said jokingly. Barry removed the small vial from his pocket. "Do you have a one cc syringe and an alcohol swab handy?"

"Let me look in my medical bag," she answered as she walked to her closet. "I'm in luck, I've got both here."

Barry walked to her desk and she handed him the syringe. He gave her the vial and she read the label. It was, as he had said, hepatitis D2 antigen. "I shall be happy to inject you if you roll up your sleeve." Sharon did as he asked and slipped off her white coat. He felt slightly jittery, and as he removed the plastic cap from the needle, he accidentally poked his own finger in his haste to withdraw the fluid from the bottle.

"Oh Barry, here's a Kleenex for your finger," said Sharon. "Is this the first time you have done this?" She laughed at his clumsiness aloud, which served to only aggravate Barry further. He was furious with himself for being so stupid as to injure himself. *It's a good thing I didn't spill any of the virus on me, or I might have sealed my own fate,* he thought. He capped the contaminated needle and placed it in his coat pocket.

"I am sorry for my clumsiness, Sharon. I'll dispose of this syringe when I get back to my clinic." He opened the wrapper of another small syringe and slowly removed the cap guard from the small 26-gauge needle, paying close attention to his task.

Barry swabbed her arm with the alcohol and withdrew 0.5 ml of the clear fluid and injected it. "There now, I knew I could do it without maiming myself," he said, laughing.

"Oh Barry, if you don't mind, leave the rest of the antigen here so I can immunize my staff. They are all terribly exposed to the virus in the clinic." Barry was startled at her request. He didn't want to leave the vial with her, but he had no grounds to refuse Sharon's innocent request. He handed her the vial and left.

After making rounds on her hospital patients and checking on her father's progress the next morning, she returned to her clinic. She informed the nurses and the secretary that she had the hepatitis antigen and impressed upon them the need for it. They didn't need convincing, since they were all aware of the high mortality rate associated with the D2 virus. Three nurses and one secretary received the antigen, but since there was still enough vaccine for five more, Sharon placed the vial in her desk drawer and returned to work. Each week, her clinic patient load increased by five more patients, and most of them were placed on the transplant list.

— 25 —

FINANCIAL PROJECTIONS

The meeting was held in the TWMC board room. David Malkin, Seymour Kramer, and James Foxworthy all sat at the long table, listening to Michael Rome's presentation.

"I am pleased to announce to you that our request for distribution of hepatitis D2 antigen has been approved. We will begin to ship the vaccine next week. In addition, the FDA has also approved our anti-rejection drug, KZ67, for distribution and sale." He smiled benevolently at the others.

"Do we have any revenue projections on either product?" asked Bently.

"Our projections indicate we will achieve sales of at least $500 million in the U.S. The rest of the world will generate in the neighborhood of $2 billion additionally, and the KZ67 sales should achieve about a half-billion dollars annually."

"That is fantastic news," said Kramer. "Financially, it comes at just the right time for us."

"I might ask at this juncture, what are the projections for the genetic transplant organs?" asked Foxworthy.

"I was about to tell you all the excellent news with regard to the organ transplant program. We have gathered all the available data from the World Health Organization, as well as specific data from many of the larger countries. In the United States, we had almost 50,000 patients awaiting organ transplants with slightly more than half of the patients dying before an organ became available. The natural growth rate for patients needing transplants has been about 25,000 new patients per year. Because of the hepatitis D2 worldwide epidemic the number of predicted potential liver transplant patients has been calculated to be 200,000 in the U.S. alone and at least another million throughout the world. We used 500,000 transplants for the world, and that brings the total number of transplant organs to 750,000 for the coming twelve-month period. At a sales price of $10,000 each, that amounts to 7.5 billion dollars."

He paused for effect. The others looked at each other in amazement at the projections. Rome then continued, "We have labs in operation already in Paris, Berlin, Rome, and England. Labs will be completed within a few months in seven other large European and Asian cities, and another in Nairobi, Kenya. We are currently negotiating with WHO for a slightly discounted rate for the poorer nations of the world. Those nations who operate in a socialistic medical environment have agreed to sign a contract with us for the organs, KZ67, and the hepatitis D2 Antigen. So then, our total sales should amount to ten billion over the next year and continue with slight declines over a five-year period. The joint venture profit will be an estimated four billion, which will be distributed quarterly to Genome, TWMC, Bently, and World Health Care. I am certain that since each one of you has a contract for bonuses tied to the bottom line of your respective companies, you shall each receive six-figure bonuses from them."

Rome smiled at each of his colleagues and basked in their accolades. He was very pleased with himself, but moreover, the thought of his ten-million-dollar bonus was soaring his spirits even higher.

~ 26 ~

BACK TO THE BASICS

"Dr. Dell, this is James Foxworthy. I am calling to inform you that Dr. James Nelson, Chief of General Surgery, is taking a sabbatical beginning tomorrow and we have not been able to provide him with a replacement. I have discussed this with the other two staff surgeons and they have each agreed to share the administration aspects and to cover the surgical call schedule a month at a time, but it would make their lives easier if you would also help in that regard. If you agree, each of you would be on call one month every three months. Your duties would, of course, be limited to patient care in the clinic and on the hospital patients. You would also be backing up the residents on call and going into surgery with them as well."

Without any reservation, Sharon agreed to help out her colleagues.

"Oh, one more thing. Can you start tomorrow? The others have previous commitments that would cause a hardship for them."

"I would be happy to do it, Mr. Foxworthy."

"I knew we could call on you, Dr. Dell. I will see that you receive appropriate compensation for your time. Thank you again." Sharon relaxed for a moment. Her father was now one week post-op and all systems were doing well. He would be out of the hospital in another week or so and was considering moving in with her for his convalescence. It was a great feeling to know he would only have to take anti-rejection drugs for two years and then would be rid of the hassles of blood tests and handfuls of pills each day. *Well,* she thought aloud, *I hope my skills in general surgery are still sharp.* She looked at the on call resident's roster for the next day and smiled when she saw Dr. Ted Evans was the resident on call. She had him paged, and he called her back promptly.

"Dr. Evans, this is Dr. Dell. I will be your backup staff surgeon tomorrow and for the next thirty days. I just wanted you to be aware there has been a change in the schedule."

"Thank you for cluing me in, Dr. Dell. I'll call you if I need help." That was the way hospital teaching programs worked. First the intern evaluated the patient, and then he called his assigned resident to confirm his impressions or to correct where he had erred. The resident was then required to call the staff surgeon on call, or in the case of a patient who already had a doctor, he was to call that designated physician. In any case, all surgeries were mandated to at least be discussed with the on call staff surgeon. Life-threatening emergencies were operated upon first and then discussed later, and, in that case, the chief resident was responsible for performing the surgery. She thought about her days when she was a resident in general surgery, and it kind of felt good to visit that place again. It was like returning home after years of being away, and she looked upon this additional change in responsibilities with eagerness. She left the hospital in an uplifted mood, feeling that her life was still very meaningful, despite the contempt she felt toward Michael Rome et al.

Sharon brewed a cup of herbal tea, then went to the bathroom for a long hot bath. This was her favorite luxury, and it wasn't often she had the time for it. Usually it was a quick shower taken on the run. After relaxing for an hour in the tub, she began to read an article in the New England Journal and fell asleep within minutes. She was abruptly startled by the annoying, rasping sound of her bedside telephone. She made a mental note to buy a new one, as she had many times in the past.

"Yes, this is Dr. Dell."

"Sorry to disturb you at this early hour—this is Dr. Evans." Sharon sat up on the side of the bed and tried to focus on the green numbers of her alarm clock. It was 5:40 in the morning. "Yes Dr. Evans, what's the problem?" she asked, trying to sound alert but knowing well she wasn't doing a convincing job at it.

"We have just admitted a twenty-four-year-old white male to the intensive care unit. He was riding a motorcycle and was hit by an auto. The chest X-ray shows a large hemothorax of the right chest with lung contusion and multiple open fractures of his fibula and tibia, as well as a displaced fracture of the femur, which is also poking through the skin. He is an insulin-dependent diabetic and has hemorrhagic shock that we are slowly overcoming with blood transfusions, but his arterial blood gasses are still poor. The reason I am calling is Dr. Swenz told his resident to get the patient ready for immediate orthopedic surgery. I don't feel it is appropriate to operate immediately in view of his shock and pulmonary insufficiency caused by the blood in the right chest impairing a contused lung from complete inflation."

Sharon, now wide awake, was rapidly evaluating all the facts. "What is Dr. Swenz's rationale for emergency surgery?"

"He told his resident he feared the development of infection from the exposed bones, and in a diabetic it might become catastrophic."

"That's true—however, it wouldn't be prudent to go in and operate right now because of the possibility of developing postoperative complications like lung collapse, adult respiratory distress syndrome, or pneumonia, any of which can be just as devastating in a diabetic patient."

"What should we do then?" asked Evans in exasperation.

"My feeling is that we wait until we are absolutely certain the hemorrhaging has stopped and his blood gases are normal. There is always the possibility that the patient has a lacerated lung or bronchus, which can happen in blunt traumatic chest injuries. By the way, have you ruled out lacerations of the spleen and liver?"

"We are in the process of CT scanning the abdomen now."

"Let's hold off on any orthopedic surgery now, and I'll see you at eight in the morning on rounds and we'll reevaluate the case. He was admitted to the general surgery service, wasn't he?" Sharon prayed that this was the case, for if the patient had been admitted to the ortho service, they would be calling the shots and it might result in the patient going to surgery now, despite her objections.

"Yes, we have been assigned the case with ortho to consult."

"Fine then, just blame me. No surgery for now. Ortho can treat conservatively for now until we stabilize him. You can start him on appropriate antibiotics and request that they insulate the wounds with appropriate dressings. You might also ask for an internal medicine consult for the diabetic management. Thank you for calling. Good night." Try as she could, there was no further sleep. Sharon tossed and turned and thought about the case. She hadn't had to exercise her clinical prowess in years, and it felt wonderful that she was able to do so with ease. She was excited and just couldn't get comfortable in her bed. Sleep was completely out of the question after an hour of staring at the ceiling and reviewing the facts of the case through her mind again and again.

At 8 a.m., Sharon was at the nurses station in the Surgical ICU, awaiting the arrival of Dr. Evans for rounds. He walked into the ICU ten minutes late, looking terrible. His hair was unruly, he needed a shave badly, and a good night's sleep wouldn't have hurt him either. She felt compassion for him, but on the other hand, this was the life of a doctor in training, and nights without sleep went with the territory. When young, you could tolerate almost anything, and although it wasn't detrimental to one's health, on occasion, it might prove to be so to the patient. This was the front line of the war waged in hospitals all over the world in their effort to overcome the legions of disease and trauma. The soldiers fought valiantly to gain the upper hand, but they never seemed to quite get there, gaining the advance in one battle and losing it in others. Each room in the hospital was a battleground within its own right and the war waged with ferocity. The newer weapons of detection and offensive warfare were pressed into service with diligence and fervor. Patients and their families offered up prayers to the Almighty in support of their doctors' efforts, but they were often unanswered. No one could answer why. Life was a mystery, albeit death often became the only solution.

She overlooked his tardiness as others had done for her while in training. "Good morning Dr. Evans," she said cheerfully.

"Good morning Dr. Dell," he replied, peering at her with droopy eyelids. "It has been a bear of a night. No sleep at all. Shall we begin with Fred Rawlins, the motorcycle verses car trauma I called you about?"

"By all means, let's start." This was the signal for the resident to present the history, examination findings, diagnosis, treatment, clinical course, and plan. When writing this in the chart, it was recorded as "soaping" the patient. The letters of the word represented *subjective* complaints, *objective* findings, *assessment* of the patient (the diagnosis), and the *plan* designed for the patient's care.

"Mr. Rawlins, an insulin-dependent diabetic since age ten, was on a motorcycle wearing a helmet when he was struck by an auto. At the moment of impact, he was catapulted to a height of about eight feet and struck the ground, landing on his chest and abdomen. On examination, he complained of numbness and tingling of the toes of the right foot, as well as chest pain. His respiratory rate was 22, pulse 140, and his blood pressure was 85 over 60. Positive pertinent physical findings included a large abrasion over the sternum with contusions of both palms and compound fractures of the right femur, distal fibula, and tibia. Abdominal and neurological exams were normal, but examination of the chest disclosed absent breath sounds over the entire right chest with dullness to percussion, both consistent with the presence of fluid. In this case, blood was suspected in view of the trauma history, but it wasn't confirmed by the chest X-ray until we repeated the chest film half an hour ago. We restored his blood pressure with blood and IV fluids, and he has remained stable in this regard until now. The orthopedists have placed his lower extremity in traction and attended to the wound dressings and IV antibiotics, while the internist has brought his sugars in control. His oxygen saturation is now normal on four liters of nasal oxygen a minute. I can't understand why we didn't see fluid in the first chest X-ray taken in the ER."

"Do you have the films here on the unit?" asked Sharon. "Yes, over here." He walked to the end of the ICU, where there were two X-ray view boxes on the wall. Sharon followed him and watched him place two films on the view box. "The one on the right is the first film."

Sharon first looked at the film from close up, and then she stood back about six feet and looked again. "What do you see?"

"It looks pretty normal to me. There's definitely no fluid

in the right pleural space." The pleural space was a potential area between the covering of the lung and the covering of the inside of the chest cavity.

"Look again and carefully compare the right to the left chest."

"Well, on second thought, there may be a suggestion of some haziness on the right as compared to the left."

"Exactly, Dr. Evans. What do you feel may be the cause of that haziness?"

"I really don't have an answer."

"Think of all the parameters that were present when the film was taken."

"The patient was on an ER gurney and the film was shot with a portable unit right there."

"Fine. Now what differences would there be if the film were taken in the X-ray department?" She loved to make her doctors solve the problem themselves and believed her job was to serve as the catalyst in the process. She could have just as easily pointed out the solution immediately, but it wouldn't have led to long-term retention. She felt the learning process was what was paramount, because it showed the budding doctors how to think.

"The patient would be standing for the X-ray in the department but would be supine in the ER."

"How did you order the film taken?"

"I asked for a stat portable of the chest."

"So you didn't specify that it should be taken with the patient sitting upright, then."

"That's correct, because the patient was still in shock and

I didn't feel it would be safe to sit him up for fear his pressure might bottom out."

"Your reasoning is sound and I would have done the same thing, but what am I alluding to?"

"You mean about the position of the patient for the film?"

"Exactly, Doctor."

"Oh, I see. If the patient is in the upright position and he has fluid in the chest, the fluid will be layered out because of gravity, and we might see a fluid line or even a dense opaqueness of the fluid itself."

"Correct. So, the fluid will be seen as dense white in nature, and above the fluid will be normal, unvisualized pleural space. Tell me then, what are we looking at in the right chest haziness?"

"Could that be the fluid, but since the patient was lying on his back the fluid is spread out in a large layer and causes the haziness instead of a white density?"

"Very well done, Dr. Evans. So you see, the blood was there all the time, you didn't see it, and therefore, you doubted your initial diagnosis. Remember, your history and examination should be corroborated by X-rays and the like. When they don't support your clinical impressions or diagnosis, look for a reason in the test you ordered, which might help explain the disparity. If necessary, repeat the test."

She was pleased with her resident's thought process. Reading portable chest films was difficult, and expertise only came with years of experience.

"I'm glad that I repeated it and that they took the film in the sitting position."

"What's the plan now?" asked Sharon.

"I'll insert a chest tube to drain the right pleural cavity of the blood."

"Good idea, and be certain to check the drainage frequently!"

"I'll do that," he affirmed. "What would your concerns be if the chest tube drainage of the blood stopped?"

"Well, the possibilities are that all the blood has been drained, the tube might be flush against the chest wall, occluding drainage from the tube orifice, or there might be clots adhering to the orifice plugging it up."

"Good answer. Keep me posted today on any further developments."

Sharon finished the rest of the rounds and headed for her office. She had a lot of paperwork to attend to and had to be in her clinic later that day. She walked to the surgical floor where her father was and visited with him for ten minutes. Seeing him walk by himself and his jaundice gone gave her pleasure. She walked out of his room and was starting for the elevators when she ran into Barry Swenz.

"Sharon, may I have a word with you please?"

"Sure you can." She sensed something was wrong. Barry looked infuriated.

"Why did you go against my orders last night on Mr. Rawlins?" he shouted. Sharon was taken aback with surprise. She had been down this route with surgical colleagues in the past. Each one had the messianic complex, and their word was law, or so they imagined, but it had always been handled with civility.

"Because I didn't want to subject the patient to surgery until he was hemodynamically stable. He was in shock due to blood loss and also in respiratory failure, you know."

"I don't need to be preached to by you or anyone else. If you recall, I am also a surgeon!"

"Then perhaps you should act like one and not a petulant little boy who didn't get his way!" Sharon was furious at her colleague's behavior.

"If he gets osteomyelitis or sepsis because of this, I will have you before the surgical committee, and you can explain it all to them!"

"Barry, you are overreacting and polarizing a situation you just haven't thought through. When you calm down, we can talk about it again, but now I'm leaving." She felt very anxious as she walked into the waiting elevator.

Barry just stood there glaring at her. After the elevator door closed, he turned and walked back toward the nurses station. His mind was overflowing with venom and hate. *That bitch, trying to make me look like a fool in front of my resident last night, I'll nail her yet.* He thought about the fact her father had audited TWMC and no doubt there would be severe repercussions from the audit. His very financial state was at stake, as well as his license to practice medicine. To boot, he was falling in debt again through his gambling addiction. That wasn't his fault. He wouldn't have had to go to Las Vegas for relaxation if the audit hadn't occurred. And who was behind it all? Sharon Dell! She'd get hers.

In the privacy of his office, behind closed doors, Barry placed a call to James Foxworthy and expressed his displeasure over the fact that Sharon had upstaged him. He insisted that she be removed from the surgical staff backup roster; this was denied by Foxworthy. Barry slammed the phone down and muttered obscenities to himself. His next call was to Michael Rome. He questioned him intensely concerning the DOC audit. Rome told him that they, as well as TWMC, hadn't heard a thing about the outcome. After he told Barry about the impending volumes of sales that were anticipated, he felt better. Rome promised he would keep Barry updated on the financial aspects, specifically when a distribution might be forthcoming to Barry according to their agreement. After he hung up, he sat back in his chair and thought about the future and what he would do with all the money he would get.

$-27-$

Adenoviruses and Oncogenes

D octors Matson and Cook were engrossed in a discussion taking place in the conference room at the Research Laboratories in Malibu. Several of the research doctors had been invited for their monthly update, which was called two weeks early because of a scientific breakthrough.

"I believe our research has proven that human cancer DNA can be injected into animals and begin to establish cancer at that site," said Paul Cook with pride. He had personally led the research for seven years and recently had a major breakthrough in the area of cancer and genetics.

"As you all know, cells of organisms must respond to environmental signals. These may be in the form of nutrients, growth factors, hormones, neurotransmitters or chemical signals. These signals control cellular growth by either activating resting cells or slowing down rapidly growing cells. The cell receives a signal, then transmits it from outside the cell into the cell, and on occasion, into the nucleus. Cells have receptors, which bind chemical signals that allow the transmission of the signal to enter the cell through the plasma cell membrane.

"You recall the discovery in 1911, whereby filtered cell free extracts from chicken tumors caused new tumors when injected into chickens. It was found that the extracts contained a virus, which caused the tumor. This was the beginning! Since the advent of recombinant DNA methodology, we have learned much. The human genome has a multitude of proto-oncogenes that can cause cancer, as well as suppressor genes that can prevent the cells from becoming malignant. A proto-oncogene is a normal cellular gene which functions in the regulation of cellular growth. It is a potential oncogene that can be induced by a signal. When this gene has been incorporated within the viral DNA, it is then called an oncogene. The signal is usually a mutation of a gene which will change the proto-oncogene to an oncogene.

"Cancer is genetic and the cancer cells are all identical, which means they are coded from the cancer cell DNA. It has been further found that all chemicals causing cancer do so by causing genetic mutation, which is to say, they damage DNA."

"We already know we can cause a normal cell to become malignant by introducing abnormal DNA into that cell," quipped Matson.

"That is correct, and in cell cultures, when normal cells are exposed to carcinogens, transformed cells are produced which have the characteristics of cancer cells and they pass these characteristics on to their daughter cells. After it was seen that certain viruses, when injected into animals, caused cancer, the race was on in genetic cancer research.

"There are two types of tumor viruses. One type has its genome within DNA, and the other in RNA. Our research has been primarily with the DNA virus types. These viruses must have the host cell's enzymes to use in their own growth and division, but some of the host cells end up with a part of the viral DNA incorporated into their own DNA and then they pass it to daughter cells in the process of cell division. This is known as the process of induction. The oncogenes carried by the virus do the transforming of the host cell through the process of encoding for oncoproteins. It is these proteins that induce the growth of the virus by stimulating host cells to grow so that it can incorporate its DNA into those cells, thereby causing the tumor. Further study led to the discovery of human oncogenes, which meant that we carried genes that could potentially kill us."

"How does the abnormal DNA or oncogene get into the vector virus?" asked Matson. "We have taken the adenovirus and, in vitro, subjected it to a living cell culture of breast cancer cells that we grew from an unfortunate patient with the disease. The virus incorporates the cancer oncogene by transduction into its own DNA. Now we have the virus acting as a carrier for the oncogene. Next, it is injected into an animal, and the viruses are trapped by the lymph nodes where they are identified as foreign and the immune system lodges its attack. The virus invades some of the lymph nodes and transmits its lethal DNA to the host cell, where it begins to produce breast cancer cells."

There was discussion among the researchers for a few minutes, and then Dr. Cook spoke.

"These results will allow researchers to develop methods to control oncoproteins and the oncogenes, and by discovering more about the systems that regulate cell growth, our therapies will be more effective. Most important is the ability we now have to produce critical cell proteins at will, and the change of their properties infers new drug strategies in the future." He sat down while everyone applauded his presentation.

"How can you be certain that the cancer from the viral oncogene is the cause and not derived from the host's own breast tissue?" asked one of the junior scientists.

"Good question! We biopsy the cancer and isolate a segment of the DNA from it. We also want a segment of the DNA that is unique to each individual, so we use the restriction fragmentation length polymorphisms method to isolate that unique segment in the recipient. The next step is to amplify the DNA with PCR and then run automatic DNA sequencers by computer. This will identify the host's DNA and compare it to the DNA of the cancer cell. If it is identical in the nucleotide sequence, it had to come from the host's cell, and if not, it came from another human cell origin."

They all knew that they were part of the advancing attack on cancer, and that made them all feel good about themselves and their work. But Matson wasn't thinking about the breakthroughs at all. He had been aware of them for quite some time, but he'd never let Cook know. It had been his custom to sneak into Cook's office each Thursday evening and read

Cook's log of experiments. Thursday was Cook's early day, and he always left at one in the afternoon, so accessing his office after five was easy. For years, Matson had followed the research advances of his colleague with envy but never realized how handy it would become. Only a few months ago, he had been asked to meet with his bosses, Michael Rome and David Malkin. They had told him they were concerned about Sharon's betrayal in calling in the DOC audit. During that meeting, they had also discussed the insertion of the microchip into her father's donor liver and the plan to execute the release of Bax protein and activate the process of apoptosis. That was when they had asked him to work along with Dr. Peter Halper. At first, he was reticent to do so; however, the additional bonus of fifty thousand dollars went a long way to change his mind. It didn't bother him to inform Halper what was going on in Cook's lab, to explain the research protocols, and to see the final product of the research—the viruses carrying the oncogenes.

~ 28 ~

THE DIAGNOSTIC PITFALL

Sharon was speaking with one of her residents in the clinic when she was interrupted by a telephone call. "Yes Dr. Evans, what's the problem with Mr. Rawlins?"

"I think you had better come to the ICU—we have a problem," he said with concern.

Sharon made a beeline for the ICU, where she found Evans at Mr. Rawlins's bedside. "Thank you for coming so soon."

"I was about to call you for an update when you called. So what has happened over the last eight hours?" she said, glancing at her watch.

"The chest tube drainage has been consistently bloody, until two-and-a-half hours ago when it suddenly changed to pure white in color."

Sharon smiled to herself in recognition of the rare complication. "What is your working diagnosis Dr. Evans?"

"I am certain the white material is chyle, which means the

patient has a chylothorax. I have obtained a positive Sudan IV stain on the fluid and the lab reports a triglyceride level of 1120 mg% on the same fluid."

"How did the fluid get into the pleural space?"

"There had to be a tear in the thoracic duct within the chest caused by the blunt trauma."

"Alright, what is the treatment plan?" She was proud of her protege's answer.

"I believe we should adopt a wait-and-see approach. There is no hurry to operate."

"Tincture of time, I agree—however, how long should we observe him before deciding to operate?"

"I don't know the answer to that. Because I have never seen this before, I did, however, go to the library and was able to review the literature."

Sharon was impressed with his desire to learn. "Tell me, what did you find?"

"Blunt trauma, as well as penetrating injuries, have been reported as well as tumors that compress or invade the thoracic duct. All the authors agree a lymph angiogram should be performed to localize the site of the leaking. In this case, the procedure should be done in one of the feet, and X-rays can be used to follow the passage of the dye into the abdominal and then the thoracic lymphatics."

"Let's return to the question of how long we should wait before surgical intervention." She widened her eyes and cocked her head to the side as if to invite a prompt answer. Receiving none, she tried a different approach to stimulate his thought process. "Always look at the positive as well as the negative aspects of a clinical decision. Often, you will be faced with a decision-making process where the decision may be right or wrong, depending on related surrounding factors of the case. Having said that, what would be the positive outcome of doing immediate surgery versus waiting?"

"I don't know of any." "Alright then, what about the negative outcome? Think of the pathological process that's happening and what effect it has on the patient."

"You mean the daily loss of the chyle from the body over a period of days?"

"Exactly! Now relate that to a negative outcome for me."

"He'll become malnourished because the fat is lost to the body, and he may develop an inability to produce antibodies as well."

"Is it worth the risk of nutritional complications and the risk of infection in a diabetic to wait and watch?"

"When you put it that way, definitely not! Especially when you consider adding the risk of acquiring a hospital-borne infection in a diabetic."

"But you see that 'putting it that way' has got to be the way you should always put it. In other words, do the risks of an action outweigh the benefits? Once you look at all clinical decisions in this light, you will be led to the correct decision and always record your rationale in the chart. It indicates that there was logical, clinically oriented thinking that went into selecting the right option for the patient. Sometimes it won't be easy, but you will always be able to identify the reasons that influence your decision process."

"That's great, Dr. Dell. It would sure be nice if they taught this type of reasoning in medical school."

"Well, that's another story. So, what are you going to do next for Mr. Rawlins?"

"I am sending him to Radiology for a stat lymph angiogram and will get him ready for surgery. I'll ask the thoracic surgeons to see him, since it will require a chest approach."

"Fine. Call me when the lymph angiogram is done. I'll be in my office for a while yet, and I'm anxious to see the films." Sharon walked from the surgical ICU directly to visit her father on the medical floor.

"Dad, you look great. You look like you are about ready to be discharged."

"I feel better each day. I can get around without the aid of a cane. I've even put on six pounds." The drains had been removed from the wound site, while the IV was still there to administer the cortisone needed to prevent any early rejection process from occurring. The KZ67 had been tested and found to be successful in preventing rejection as long as steroids were administered for at least thirty months. There always loomed the possibility that the body's immune system might uncover some minor change and start to reject the transplanted organ. This was theoretical, however, because it had never been found to occur. Sharon sat and chatted with her dad about world events and politics. Karl told her he was ready to leave the hospital, and the sooner the better, but Sharon convinced him to allow the medical doctors to make that decision. She returned to her office and attacked the piles of letters and documents on her desk.

Before she knew it, two hours had flown by and her phone rang. "Yes, Dr. Evans, I'll meet you in Radiology." She scrambled out of the office and entered the elevator, riding it to the basement. Evans met her at the reading room with an air of excitement.

"What's the verdict?" asked Sharon. "Look at these films." He had a pile of X-ray film in his hand. The radiologist had gone home after reviewing the films with Evans. He placed a view of the abdomen onto the view box. The radio-opaque dye was easily seen arising from the pelvis into the abdomen all within the lymphatic channels. There, suddenly, at about the T-12 level, which was high in the abdomen, the dye was seen extravasating from the area of the abdominal lymphatic duct known as the cisterna chyli. The dye spilled over into the area below the right diaphragm.

"The rupture is in the abdominal lymphatics and not in the thorax," said Sharon, amazed.

Taking a cue, Evans placed a second film on the view box. The chest showed there was free dye within the right pleural space, which could also be seen in the chest tube situated posteriorly.

"Amazing," she muttered. "How do you explain this, Dr. Evans? We were thinking the patient had a tear in the thoracic duct, and there is none to be seen there. There is, however, a large tear in the abdominal lymphatics at the cisterna, with dye in the right subphrenic space."

"The only answer I can offer is that we know there is an abdominal leak and the thoracic duct is open and picking up the dye from above the diaphragm. The only plausible answer is that there must be a rent in the diaphragm that is allowing dye to move from the peritoneal cavity to the pleural cavity. Furthermore, the reason the chest tube was draining the chyle was that it has to be located at the rent in the diaphragm so it is suctioning directly from the abdominal peritoneal cavity and not from the pleural cavity."

Sharon was nodding her head in agreement and laughing aloud. This was one of those things that happened every so often in medicine, the kind that boggled the mind and were what really made medicine so fascinating. The haphazard placement of a chest tube over a hole in the diaphragm led them all to believe the thoracic duct was leaking, when it really was the cisterna chyli located in the abdominal lymphatics. She told Evans to alert the chest surgeons they would not be needed and to call the general surgeons right away.

Surgery went very well. Abdominal exploration was performed and the cisterna was repaired. A rent in the posterior portion of the right leaf of the diaphragm was also found and repaired. After surgery, Evans realized if he had waited, the duct would have never healed itself but moreover, he had learned a valuable lesson in medicine. Even if you are absolutely certain of a diagnosis, there must always be room to consider a diagnostic pitfall, and even then, circumstances may hide the real answer.

-29-

LYMPHADENOPATHY

Sharon was tired. Operating five days a week to keep up with the backload of transplant patients was taking its toll on her. During the past four weeks, the number of children requiring liver transplants had been increasing drastically, but on this morning, she had about an hour to herself before the next surgery was scheduled to begin.

"Dr. Dell, may I speak with you for a moment?" asked Ginny Ross. She had worked as a clerk in the transplant clinic for six years.

"Sure, Ginny, come on in and sit down," replied Sharon, somewhat relieved to take a break from her routine. "What can I do for you?"

"I need your advice. I noticed something hard in my right armpit a week ago," she said solemnly.

Sharon became alert and her eyes widened. "Have you gone to your own doctor about this?"

"No, I haven't. I've been scared to! I trust you, Dr. Dell. Will you examine me, please?" she pleaded with moist eyes.

Sharon went to Ginny and took her hand. "Of course I will. Come along with me."

They walked together from her office to the clinic.

"Karen, please place Ginny in an examining room and gown her for a breast examination."

"Of course. Ginny, come with me, I'll fix you up." Ginny followed with tears in her eyes.

Sharon walked into the small room with a large clipboard. "I want to take your history first," she said with a smile. "How old are you, Ginny?"

"I am thirty-two."

"Any children?"

"Yes, two."

"Tell me, is there a history of breast cancer in your family?"

"No, my mother and three sisters have never had it."

"Do you take any medicines or hormones at all?"

"No, I don't."

"Have your menstrual cycles been normal?"

"Yes."

"How much coffee do you drink?" Sharon was hoping she would find fibrocystic breast disease, which could be aggravated by large amounts of coffee.

"One cup in the morning."

"Have you had breast pain before your periods?"

"Sometimes I do, but it's not bad."

"How long have you been performing breast self-examinations?"

"I have been doing it for a couple years."

"Have you ever felt any other lumps during this time?"

"No, never!"

"Has the skin in your breast been red or tender?"

"No."

"Have you had any red skin or infection in your armpit, arm, or hand in the last few weeks?"

"No." "Have you cut yourself while shaving the area?"

"No."

"Okay. Ginny, please lie down on the table." Sharon examined her patient methodically. She placed her hand in Ginny's right armpit, or axilla as it was more properly known, and palpated the area. Immediately she was aware of a three-centimeter firm mass that was not tender. The skin appeared normal, and there was no evidence of local infection.

"Ginny, I want you to have a mammogram and an ultra sound of the axilla right away."

"Fine with me. I'm really nervous about this."

"Look, this may only be an enlarged lymph node, but I can't be certain until we get the tests back. My examination did not reveal any masses in the breasts, and that is a good sign. Usually, when there is a metastatic spread of breast cancer to a lymph node, there is a palpable breast mass as well. I'll call you after I see the results of the mammogram and ultrasound later today."

"Thank you, Dr. Dell."

Sharon walked to the OR thinking about Ginny. *I don't like the feel of that lymph node. It felt too hard to be a benign enlargement. I sure hope I'm wrong though.* She tried to put it out of her mind and concentrate on the upcoming surgery.

The surgery concluded at 4 p.m., and Sharon made a bee-line for the Radiology Imaging Department. "Dr. Simpson, how are you?" she asked with a big smile.

"I'm fine, and you?"

"Just a bit overworked and tired. I wonder if you have had a chance to look at the mammogram and axillary lymph node ultrasound on Ginny Walters?"

"I just dictated my findings. The mammogram was completely normal, but I'm afraid I have bad news on the ultrasound of the lymph nodes. The nodes look like malignancy." Sharon sighed deeply and shook her head slowly. It was hard for a doctor when the reality of cancer was confronted involving a patient, but it was twice as bad when it was a friend or family member.

At last she spoke. "This is very strange. If it is breast cancer, one would expect to find the primary by mammography, unless it is a lymphoma or some rare tumor."

"You are correct," offered Dr. Simpson. "Head and neck cancers, or even lung, might be the source. It would be unusual for a lymphoma to arise in only one area of lymph nodes."

"Let's do a workup tomorrow. A CT of the chest and abdomen, for starters."

"It might be a good idea to do a Sestamibi Scan on her breast. That's our latest tool for breast cancers."

"Tell me about it."

"Well, it's a potassium nuclear isotope, which has an affinity for breast cancer. We inject it and then scan the breast. If it shows up on the scan, it is ninety-eight percent conclusive. In

Europe, they are doing away with many of the breast biopsies that were being done for suspicious lumps."

"Fine, go ahead and do it." Sharon walked to the elevator and went to her office.

She was unhappy about the fact that she was about to begin a week's vacation with her dad. Sharon picked up the hospital directory and opened the section on oncology. She found what she was looking for and dialed Michael Herbert's extension. She had been attracted to his good looks and the fact that he was single at the age of thirty-six. In addition, he was also very personable and intelligent. He stood six feet and weighed 180 pounds, with blue eyes and long blond hair. She picked up the phone and dialed his number.

"Michael, this is Sharon," she said, feeling a warm flush spread over her face. *I'm glad I'm doing this on the phone rather than in person*, she quipped to herself.

"How are you, Sharon?"

"I'm fine, but I have a favor to ask."

"Sure, what is it?"

"My clinic clerk, Ginny Ross, asked me to examine her today because she was concerned about a mass in her right axilla. I found a three-centimeter, very hard mass, but the rest of the exam including the breast, was normal. She really has no risk factors and her family history was negative. The mammogram was normal, but the ultrasound of the nodes were interpreted by Dr. Simpson as probably malignant."

"That's horrible! How may I assist you?"

"I'm scheduled for a week's vacation beginning in two days, so I would like you to assume Ginny's care tomorrow.

I wanted to work her up completely before I referred her to you, but that will be impossible on this short notice."

"I would be delighted. Have her come to my office tomorrow at two."

"That will be great. She should have completed the CT scans and the Sestamibi Scan of the breast by then."

"Call me when you return from vacation." She thought she picked up a hidden message in his request. No, she was only wishing! She then left for home.

Her dad had been living with her temporarily since his discharge from the hospital six weeks ago, and he was now back to normal.

"Hi Dad, it's T minus two days."

"I can't wait. I have always wanted to fish Canada for northern pike, but never had the opportunity to do so. What a birthday present you've given me, I can't believe it. One whole week of fishing in Saskatchewan Province."

"Actually we are going about 150 miles north of Saskatoon." She busied herself preparing a light dinner while she conversed.

"That country is all water and no people anywhere."

"We'll fly to the fishing camp by seaplane, Dad."

"I love it! I'm as excited as I used to get when you were a little girl and we would go fishing."

"Me too. You know how I love to fish!"

"They will have all the tackle there, right?"

"I told you that twice already. Don't you believe me?"

"Of course I do. I just don't want to get there and find that I don't have anything to fish with."

Sharon threw her arms around her dad and kissed him on the cheek. "Stop worrying!" she scolded. "Make sure you pack some warm clothes as well as your rain gear. June in Canada can be nasty."

"I'm already packed. One duffle bag for me, and how many for you, my dear?" he asked raising his eyebrows.

"One, only one!

"Thank God you don't take after your mother in that regard. She would have taken at least three bags of clothes and one of creams and jellies for her face and skin," he replied with misty eyes. Sharon saw his sadness and moved quickly to change the subject. "Have you ever fished for walleye or lake trout, Dad?"

His face lit up. "No, I haven't but I'm looking forward to it now!"

"Let's eat now," she said as she placed a plate of food in front of him.

The following morning, Sharon went to her clinic to speak with Ginny. "I have arranged for Dr. Michael Herbert to take over your care, Ginny."

"Are you giving up on me?"

"No, certainly not. I'm going fishing with my dad for a week. I would have referred you to him when I had finished working you up, because the mammogram was normal, but the ultrasound is suspicious for a tumor. I have ordered further studies in radiology this morning. Please get there by ten o'clock. They may ask you to return in the afternoon for more testing, but your appointment with Dr. Herbert is at two this afternoon, so let radiology know." She saw a tear form in Ginny's eye. "Everything will be alright, I'm sure of it." Sharon talked with her patient for an hour, and her compassion allayed Ginny's fears.

"Thank you so much, Dr. Dell. I feel better now."

"May I speak with you, Dr. Dell," interrupted the charge nurse of her clinic, Gail Poland.

"Come on in, Ginny is just on her way to radiology."

"Dr. Dell, have you got a minute to feel something?"

"Sure, what do you want me to feel?"

"I just noticed this enlarged lymph node in my right axilla!"

"What? How long have you had it?"

"I just became aware of it this morning." Sharon's mind was racing. *How could this happen a second time in a few days?*

"Slip off your blouse, Gail, and place your right arm on my shoulder." Sharon placed her hand in Gail's axilla and palpated the area.

"You have a one-and-one-half centimeter firm node here. Is it tender?"

"No."

Sharon took a detailed history from Gail and led her into an examination room, where she completed her physical examination. She couldn't believe it. The findings were the same as Ginny's. She wrote a lengthy note on a clean sheet of paper.

"I want you to have some testing done immediately!"

"Do you think it might be malignant?"

"I don't know, Gail."

"Look, Dr. Dell, I know what's going on with Ginny's. We're close friends." At that point, Sharon felt more ease in discussing her concerns, because she would not be violating patient confidentiality.

"Tell me what you know about Ginny's case."

Gail gave the details of Ginny's medical problems without missing a beat.

"Since you do know her condition, I must tell you I am baffled by this. In medicine, they say, diseases comes in threes. You are the second case in two days to present to me with the exact same history and physical findings."

"What does that mean?"

"I can't put it all together now, but I promise you I will. I want you to go to radiology and have them do these studies." She wrote her requests for mammogram, Sestamibi scan of the breast, and CT scans of the chest and abdomen on her prescription pad and handed them to Gail. "By the way, Gail, you are aware that I will not be here next week?"

"I know, you are on vacation."

"I want you to follow up with Dr. Herbert in my absence. I will alert him that you will call."

"Thank you, I will. Have a great vacation—you really deserve it, Dr. Dell." She hugged her.

– 30 –

AFTER THE BIG ONES

Karl and Sharon were seated comfortably on Northeast Flight 330 out of LAX bound for Milwaukee where they were to board a connecting flight to Saskatoon.

"Tell me Sharon, how long is the layover in Milwaukee?"

"It's about three hours, Dad. We will arrive in Saskatoon at nine this evening and spend the night there. We fly out at six a.m. to Lac LaRonge and hop the seaplane to the fishing camp."

"How long is the flight to Lac LaRonge?"

"Less than an hour, and the seaplane flight leaves as soon as we get there."

The plane landed in a rain storm, and upon arriving at the terminal gate, they were informed that their flight had been delayed for two hours because of the storm.

"Are you hungry, Sharon?"

"As a matter of fact, I am." Karl looked at his daughter wearing a baseball cap, Levis, and a sweat shirt, and swore she was still a teenager. She was one of those fortunate females who always looked less than twenty, no doubt a genetic trait from her mother, he surmised. He was well aware of the many glances from men who also were admiring the fresh California scenery. They walked the small airport ramps in short order and rapidly determined the restaurants and shops closed at sundown, leaving a McDonald's as the only place to stave off the hunger pangs. Karl looked at her and shrugged his shoulders with outstretched palms. Sharon laughed and accompanied him to the line. They each feasted on a quarter pounder with cheese, fries, and Diet Cokes. A Midwest airport was definitely not the place to do serious people-watching but was much more conducive to promoting a nap, which they both took part in upon their return to the departure gate. By the time the flight left, it was already 10 p.m., which put them into Saskatoon at eleven and their hotel by midnight.

The next morning at 5:30 they were on the way back to the airport to catch the six o'clock flight to Lake LaRonge. Arriving there at 6:40, they found their way to the seaplane shuttle a short mile away. In no time, they were bound for the Paull River Camp aboard the *Twin Sea Otter*. The wide vista below revealed nothing but water and greenery from the air. The waterways seem to connect miraculously amid land masses of all sizes and shapes. They flew north for 150 miles, put down on the Paull River, and taxied to the small dock where they were met by Sam the proprietor, his assistant Jack, and their Indian guide, Joe. Both Sharon and Karl were feeling jubilant, and their faces gave them away as they were led to their cabin.

"You folks are real lucky to be here at this time," said Sam.

"Really? Why is that," answered Karl.

"Because the other folks canceled, so you are the only ones here."

"How many people do you take at one time?" asked Sharon.

"We have five cabins which will accommodate three to four in each, but I never book more than ten people a week."

"I guess it must be difficult to tend to a herd of fishing nuts," said Karl. "The problem is there's always a bunch of heavy drinkers. They bring along large supplies of liquor and drink nonstop for a week. I warn them that I won't take them on the water if they drink, and I never allow them to take any more than a few beers apiece into the boat."

"That sounds like a reasonable solution to me," said Karl.

"It's to protect my Indian guides as well. I don't want them to drink on the job, for all the obvious reasons."

"What tribe are the Indians from?" asked Sharon.

"They're Cree Indians. They have inhabited these lands for hundreds of years; many have intermarried with the Canadians."

"How is the fishing?" she asked with enthusiasm.

"Funny you should ask," answered Sam with a twinkle in his eye. "The walleye fishin' has been great, the jack even greater, but the lake trout have been spotty."

"What are jack?" asked Karl.

"That's what we call the great northern pike up here."

"Okay, thanks for the education. Now tell me about the lake trout. How do we fish for them here?"

"Here's the pitch, folks," answered Sam. "The Canadian

Government has given me charge of eight miles of the Paull River and six large lakes. These are assigned to me only. I must tell you that it is impossible to get to fish everything in one week. One of the lakes is great for lake trout. The lakes have just thawed a month ago, and for the rest of June the trout are spawning and remain near the surface. We troll for them with spoons or any other crankbait that doesn't run deep. You are limited to three trout apiece each day."

"How large are they?" asked Sharon.

"They average about three pounds, and they are some fighting fish," he hastened to add.

"What about the 'jack'?" asked Karl.

"They are all over here, but we have one lake that produces trophy fish."

"How big do they come?" asked Sharon.

"Trophy fish are all over fifteen pounds and can go as much as twenty-five."

"Wow, that would be some catch," she retorted.

Sam took them on a tour of the facilities located on a three-acre parcel. The log cabins were situated high on the river's bank, and inside they were very rustic. Accommodations included a kitchen table with a wood-burning stove and two bedrooms with bunk beds. The kitchen also had a rustic sink, while the outhouse was located a hundred feet away in the midst of the forest next to an enclosed shower stall. Electricity was provided by a diesel generator that was turned on at six in the morning and shut off at 10 p.m.

"This is beautiful," said Sharon aloud.

"It sure is," agreed Karl. "No television, radio or newspapers; only the sounds of nature."

"Breakfast is at seven and dinner at six. Shore lunches are provided daily from the fish you catch in the morning. Joe will see to the lunches daily. It's almost noon. Why don't you get ready to go fishin' and I'll rustle up some sandwiches that you can take out with you?"

"Fine, we'll meet you at the dock in twenty minutes," said Karl.

"Why not ten?" said Sharon as she laughed at her father. "Can't you get into fishing clothes in less than twenty minutes, Dad?"

"I was only thinking of you, dear. I wanted to give you time to fix your makeup for the fish," he replied with sincerity.

"I'll bet that I beat you to the dock." She quickly made tracks back to the cabin.

In less than ten minutes, Sharon was at the dock, talking to Joe and awaiting her father's arrival.

"I don't believe you beat me," Karl said as he approached the dock.

"Sure did, Dad. I don't have time to waste when I'm going fishing."

"You folks can come aboard now," said Joe. He was about five-and-a-half feet tall, two hundred pounds, and had coal-black hair, dark eyes, and a ruddy complexion. Karl and Sharon took their seats in the aluminum skiff, which was powered by a 35-HP Johnson outboard.

The water was calm and there was no wind while the sun peeked through a high, scattered cloud layer.

It took ten minutes for them to arrive at the first fishing spot on the river. The current was about four knots, and they anchored about twenty feet from shore. Joe took a rod and set the line up with a yellow-colored jig. "Throw this over and when you hit bottom move it around slowly."

He attached a white jig to the other line and handed it to Karl. "Cast it on the right side of the boat and slowly retrieve the line."

He then threw his own line over the side and waited.

"I got one!" shouted Sharon, as she reeled in her line. The tip of the bent pole jumped about erratically while Sharon began to laugh and talk aloud to herself. "Come on now, don't let go." The fish was hauled aboard and she beamed as she held it up for her father to admire.

"That's about a two-pound walleye, Miss," said Joe, with all the excitement of a person who had just been informed he had underpaid his income taxes.

"Sharon, that's a great fish," said Karl just as his pole bent over. "I've got one too!" Karl landed a smaller although very respectable walleye. The fish continued to bite, and at four o'clock Joe announced that they were returning to the camp. In the fish box were more than twenty walleye, and none weighed less than a pound. They returned to camp and prepared for an early dinner.

Later that evening, they sat outside and looked at the sky. At 10 p.m., it was still light, which continued until 2 a.m. Darkness followed for about two hours, and then it was light all over again. This was the way it was in northern Canada. The northern lights were visible only during July and August, so they were not afforded that luxury. The temperature at night was about 60 degrees and there was no humidity at all, but there were mosquitoes en masse.

The following morning found Karl sipping coffee at the river's bank at six. He had risen very early and was excited about the forthcoming day. After a hearty breakfast of muffins and eggs, they were again on the boat with Joe, headed for places unknown. He went south for an hour and then entered a small canal about twenty feet wide. They followed it a mile or so and found themselves at the end of the waterway, which had been obstructed by a dam of freshly cut timber.

"These beavers are very busy, as you can see," said Joe.

"How long ago do you think this dam was built?" asked Sharon.

"Two days ago we cleared the dam, and they have completely rebuilt it," he answered as he leaped out of the boat and onto the dam to clear the tree limbs. In just a few minutes, the water flowed freely into the large lake. As they entered the vast body of water, they saw nothing but the lake surrounded by trees. It was an immense lake with an occasional small island harboring dense foliage rising out of the water. Bald eagles were plentiful, soaring in pairs, also eager to demonstrate their fishing abilities while the sun shone brightly, warming the occupants of the boat as it sped toward one of the islands. Joe reduced the engine to trolling speed and handed a rod to Sharon.

"Put a rattletrap on the end of this line," he grunted. "We'll troll for trout." Sharon opened her tackle box and withdrew the glistening, shiny, half-ounce lure shaped and artistically designed like a big-eyed small bait fish. She held it up next to her ear and shook it twice. "Those BBs are still there," she said to Karl.

Karl smiled as he gazed upon his daughter. He recalled the slight disappointment when she was born because he had wished so hard for a son to take fishing. Little had he ever dreamed that a girl could be as good a fisherman as a boy. Here was the proof of the pudding sitting right in front of him, wearing the baseball cap, being very serious about the task before her. Yes indeed, he thought, she was a better fisherman than he was. Her tackle box contained every sort of lure and device known to man, and this was only her freshwater lure-box. She also was an avid saltwater sports fisherman, and every chance she got would fish for different species. Never had she ever demonstrated any squeamishness about baiting a hook when she was first learning the sport. She had mastered the spinning reel and was able to place a lure on any target within fifty yards with deadly accuracy while Karl had grown up with the standard bait casting reel. He was every bit as proud of these abilities as he was of her surgical prowess because he believed in being well-rounded in the real world. He hated the bookworm, grinds, or nerds as they were currently referred to. In his experience, he had observed that most of the nerds were ineffectual as deliverers of good medical care.

"Well, are you going to get your line wet?" she asked.

"Oh … I was daydreaming." He placed a yellow spoon with a white tail feather on his line and let it out over the stern. They both were intent on watching their lines.

"Hold it, Joe!" shouted Karl. "I've got one." His pole was bent 30 degrees and the line snapped taut as the tip of the rod danced with excitement. Karl fought the fish with expertise, and when it surfaced next to the boat for a moment to feign exhaustion, Karl muttered something about, "Now I've got ya." But he was sadly duped as the trout headed for deep six in a hurry. Karl reset the drag on the reel to allow the fish his head in a reflex action so as not to snap the six-pound test monofilament line. After repeating the scenario again, he finally landed the fish.

"He's just under five pounds," said Joe, while holding the fish up for Sharon to capture on film. Karl then held the trophy while she took another shot.

"What a battle!" exclaimed Karl.

"You did good, Dad!" she responded as she cast her line out again. It seemed that just as it hit the water, the Rattletrap was devoured by a fish who was just waiting for the opportunity. She expertly played it to the boat and Karl netted it for her.

Joe looked at it flopping in the net and said, "Two-and-a-half pounds." Karl looked at his daughter and remarked that she would have to do a lot better to catch up with him.

That was how the hours passed on the lake. They would joke and prod each other's fishing ability. At noon, Joe announced they would have lunch and headed his craft toward the island. After tying up the boat, they gathered wood and started a fire while Joe cleaned the fish. The fish carcasses were thrown into the water, which served as a lunch announcement for the circling fowl. In short order, the fish were spiked through with green wood and allowed to roast on the fire while cans of creamed corn were heating on the hot rocks at the fire's base. Eventually they feasted upon a succulent pink lake trout with corn and fried onions. It was a scrumptious feast for the three hungry sportsmen. The rest of the afternoon was spent in the lake, catching and releasing lake trout. Sharon stopped counting after the fourteenth fish was caught. They headed back to the camp well satisfied and fulfilled with their first exposure to Canadian lake trout fishing; it was much more than either had expected.

On the way back to camp, Joe decided to have one last whack at the walleye. Everyone rigged up with rapalas and began to cast and retrieve for the wary fish. In a few moments, Sharon announced casually that she had one on. "He's a good-sized one!"

Then Karl shouted that he too had hooked one. They both retrieved their lines, and when the fish was next to the boat, both of them were dumfounded to see that the walleye had two rapalas in his mouth. The fish was brought aboard and Joe told them, "This was a hungry fish."

"I have never seen a fish bite two lures and be caught with both of them still in his mouth," said Karl. Just then, the fish shook itself violently and managed to stick Sharon with one of the exposed hooks hanging from the walleye's mouth.

"Ow! He stabbed me," screamed Sharon. She squeezed her finger and encouraged the bleeding. "I guess I'm lucky the hook didn't remain in the finger," she said.

"Here, let me see that," said Karl. "It looks clean. You'll be all right."

"Well then, Dad, whose fish really is it?" She then burst into a laughing fit that became so contagious both Joe and Karl joined in for a long while.

The following morning, their guide headed north to a point where the river seemed to end at a waterfall. Beaching their boat, they carried their gear across a hundred yards of forest trail onto another beach, which was located on yet another large lake. They spent the morning jigging for walleye and the afternoon fishing for the great northern pike in the *trophy* lake. In a matter of minutes, each of them began to catch fish that ranged between seven and ten pounds. It seemed as though a fish was caught on every cast, but only half of them were boated and then released. Sharon began to complain that her right arm and shoulder were tired from all the activity. Karl laughed at her comments. Suddenly, her line snapped taut and the pole achieved a perfect U shape. "I've got a big one!" she screamed while playing the monster. She readjusted the reel drag to lessen the tension so as not to snap the line. The fish then surfaced about thirty feet from the boat, and all three of them screamed. That was the first time Joe had shown any excitement. "Don't lose it, don't lose it!" he cried, while Karl was offering suggestions to Sharon as the fish headed for deep water again.

"He's got to be at least twenty five pounds!" shouted Karl.

"I believe it, Dad," she shouted back, laughing. Sharon stood up in the center of the boat, trying to follow the fish's direction as it zigzagged from side to side. Ten minutes later, the fish was netted by Joe. He grunted as he pulled the flopping creature aboard. Quickly, he laid a measuring tape along its side and announced, "Fifty inches!" Just as quickly, he weighed the fish and proclaimed, "Twenty-seven pounds. Sharon, come here and hold the fish while Karl takes pictures."

Karl shot four pictures rapidly and Joe placed the big fish back in the water. Karl and Sharon saw that the fish was lying tilted on its side at a 30-degree angle on the water surface. "He's not dead, is he?" she asked with sincerity.

"No. Watch this resuscitation technique," replied Joe. He grabbed the fish just in front of the tail and pushed the monster forward a few feet. He continued to repeat the procedure while Sharon and Karl both looked on with concern.

"The water will go through the gills and he will be fine in a minute," announced Joe.

"Are you sure?" she asked with reservation. "Trust me, I've been doing this for many years." No sooner had he muttered those words when the giant jack began to wiggle his tail and remain at 90 degrees to the water. Joe let loose of the fish, and it quickly swam away from the boat. They all breathed a sigh of relief that the fish was okay and would return to its home to produce more of its own kind for others to enjoy the thrill of catching.

During the rest of the day, they caught more fish than they had ever in their lives. This was truly a paradise. The fish were rarely bothered by intruders, so their appetites were ferocious. Every two casts produced a fish that was landed in the boat, and Karl caught a twenty-one pounder as well. They were having the time of their lives enjoying the outdoors and each other's company. Sharon was conscious of an uncomfortable feeling in her right armpit, but chalked it off to mild lymph node enlargement secondary to the finger wound sustained from the fish hook the day before.

The rest of the fishing for the remaining four days were just as fruitful. No matter where they went to fish, it continued to be fantastic. By the last day, they were all fished out.

"I don't ever remember catching so many fish," Sharon said.

"Me either."

"My right arm is hurting me from all the fishing."

"Take a Motrin."

"That's a good idea, do you have any with you?"

"I'll get some for you when we get back to camp." After dinner, Sharon swallowed two Motrin tablets and went to sleep.

The next morning found them on the Sea Otter headed south to Lac La Ronge, then to Saskatoon and Milwaukee, then finally to LAX. All the way home, Sharon kept rubbing her shoulder, professing her discomfort and attributing it to all the fishing activity combined with the finger wound. The trip was tiresome but uneventful, and they were home by 10 p.m. California time.

~31~

TWMC RECEIVES
A VISITOR

Bright and early the following morning, Sharon was at her desk attempting to sort her mail. At long last, she had managed to reduce the stack to a manageable size, and now she opened the remaining letters. She was interested in the reports from Michael Herbert, her oncology colleague. Rapidly reading through the two-page summary on Ginny (Virginia) Ross, she saw that a fine needle biopsy of the lymph nodes had been read out by the pathologist as breast carcinoma with metastasis to the axillary lymph nodes. Sharon sighed in sadness over the diagnosis and picked up the second report on Gail Poland. Scanning the first page, she rapidly went to the end of the report. Oh, my God!" she said aloud, startling herself to hear her own voice. She reached for the phone and dialed Michael Herbert.

"Michael, I have just read your reports on Ginny and Gail. What is going on?"

"I know, it's unbelievable, isn't it?"

"Two employees with metastatic breast cancer and in the same place?"

"It's uncanny, and I can't even come close to explaining it."

"There must be something in common here." Sharon struggled for a reasonable explanation to account for two women having axillary lymph nodes with breast cancer occurring at the same time, but was left with a blank.

"The really strange feature is that neither one of them has a cancer in the breast by any of the testing we have done. That is rarer than hen's teeth!"

"What bothers me Michael is the old adage that these things always come in threes."

"You're right, I hate to think about that."

"Well, what's the treatment plan?"

"I have sent the tissue for genetic analysis. Once I get the results, I will be in a better position to suggest the best treatment option."

"Fine, let's keep in touch."

"Say, on that note, how about letting me take you to dinner on Friday evening?"

"Uh … why yes," she said, "I would love it. I'll talk to you again before then." That was an unexpected surprise.

▲ ▲ ▲

Karl received the Fedex from the Sacramento DOC office. He was instructed to continue the audit on TWMC placed on a temporary hold a few months ago. As he methodically reviewed the data before him, he quickly realized that no-where in the medical charts was there any evidence that an anti-rejection drug other than steroids had been used to treat the postoperative transplant patients. He did note, however, that these patients had all been treated with something called KZ67. He knew enough about hospital bylaws that mandated any approved research drug be designated as such and ap-propriate informed consent be obtained from each patient before the drug was used. None of the charts contained these consents, and it was also strange that only one doctor cared for these patients. Dr. Barry Swenz, an orthopedist, was the only one who ever saw them, no matter what organ had been transplanted into the patient. On that note, Karl thought he had better inform his boss at the DOC of his findings. "Hello, John, this is Karl. I must speak with you about some irregularities I've found in the records of TWMC."

"What have you got?" replied John Higgins, the medical director of the DOC.

"The records all have a similar pattern. The patients that came for a repeat organ transplant were covered by World Health Care HMO and were all taking something recorded as KZ67. There are no informed consents for the drug, and re-gardless of the transplanted organ, the patients were all cared for by one orthopedic physician. In addition, the only other drug these patients were taking was Prednisone for about two years, and then it was stopped. All the repeat transplants occurred be-tween the thirty-sixth and fortieth month after the first one."

"My God, what's going on there? This is a quality issue that needs immediate intervention by our office. Can you get me your reports by the end of the week? I'll review them and contact the Attorney General's office in order to obtain an immediate TRO."

"I'll do my best to help you get that restraining order, John. What do you think about my interviewing Dr. Swenz?"

"Good idea. Get as much information as you can."

"Fine then, I'll get right on it!" Karl hung up the phone and called TWMC, arranging an appointment with Dr. Swenz for the next afternoon.

He arrived at TWMC earlier than his scheduled appointment with the idea he would surprise Sharon and perhaps have lunch with her. He rode the elevator to the sixth floor and headed for her office. Walking into the secretary's office, he motioned for her not to reveal his presence while he peeked into Sharon's office. She was busy with paperwork when he cleared his throat. She looked up and beamed. "Dad, what are you doing here?" She got up and hastened to hug him.

"I've come to take you to lunch so we can talk about these pictures I have."

"What pictures?" In a few days at work, she had all but forgotten the fishing trip.

"Canada … fishing."

"Of course, I've been so busy I haven't had time to think about the wonderful time we had."

"I know, that's why I'm here to remind you with the pictures."

"Great, I'm starved. Let's go."

Karl followed Sharon to the elevator where they

descended to the first floor and entered the cafeteria. "I just love hospital food, don't you?" asked Karl.

"It staves off the hunger, but you've got to use your imagination when you eat."

"Like what?"

"Like pretend it's really good."

"Nummy, yummy." Karl grimaced as he bit into the egg salad sandwich. "Too much mayo."

Sharon laughed at her father. He was always a finicky eater, and on more than one occasion she had witnessed him voicing his displeasure over a gastronomical creation. "It's only a sandwich, but you can pretend it's a Wolfgang Puck pizza, if you want." They continued small talk for a while, and when they had concluded lunch, Karl handed the pictures to Sharon. She was exuberant as she studied each photo and summarized each one to Karl, who just loved every minute of it. "Well, I have to get to clinic, Dad. Thanks for lunch. I'll see you later tonight at home." She started to walk away from him, but suddenly turned around as though forgetting something. "I forgot to ask you, Dad, are you here on business?"

"Yes, I am. I have an appointment with Dr. Swenz in about twenty minutes." Sharon was stunned and nodded as she walked away from the table.

Karl sipped his coffee and then walked to the elevator. He was thinking of the time he was a medical resident as he noticed the many doctors scurrying about. He was impressed over the fact that now there were many more women in medicine, whereas in his time, there were ten males to every female.

Exiting on the fourth floor, he found his way to Dr. Swenz's office and announced himself to the secretary. In short order, she ushered him into the inner office where Dr. Swenz walked around his desk with an outstretched hand to greet his visitor. "So glad to make your acquaintance, Dr. Dell. Please have a seat." He gestured to the chair situated to the right of his desk.

"I won't waste your time, Dr. Swenz. I'll get right to the point."

"Please do. I don't have the slightest idea why you are here."

"The DOC has charged me with investigating TWMC with regard to the treatment of organ transplant patients. In that regard, I have conducted a medical chart audit, and as a result, I have some questions to ask you."

"That's fine."

"Tell me Doctor, why are you the only physician who does the post-op transplant follow-up care on these patients?"

"I have been trained in the method and science of taking care of these patients."

"But you are an orthopedist, and many of these cases belongs in the realm of internal medicine or pediatrics, not orthopedics."

"They all require similar treatment to prevent rejection of their transplanted organs. It's only a matter of adjusting drug dosage and following lab tests for signs of rejection."

"You're not proficient in, nor have you had training in, these specialties outside of orthopedics. I have discussed this issue with the Medical Board of California and they also are of the same opinion."

"Well, I strongly differ in that opinion, Dr. Dell. I believe that first and foremost a doctor cares for the whole patient, not only his area of specialty."

"A good doctor will always look at the patient as a whole being but will also know his limitations," responded Karl in a failed attempt at stating the obvious. "Specifically, he should realize when he has no training in certain areas and, therefore, should refer the patient to the most appropriate specialist. Just because the California medical license says physician and surgeon on it, it should not be misconstrued to mean that all licensees are surgeons in the true sense of the word. A surgeon must demonstrate competence through his residency training."

Swenz was quickly becoming irritated with Karl.

"Look, there was no one else to follow these patients, and I agreed to do it."

"Who did you make that agreement with?"

"Uh, I don't think that's any of your business!" shouted Swenz.

Karl realized that he'd struck a nerve. "I was only attempting to understand how it was that all the patients you cared for after transplant surgery belonged to World Health Care HMO?" Swenz became red-faced and taunted Karl. "I suppose your righteous daughter put you up to all this. Well, you don't know anything, and neither does Sharon. She ought to mind her own business about things that don't concern her!"

"Doctor, I am not trying to be argumentative. I am only trying to understand the facts concerning these patients. If you won't help me now, I can assure you that the medical board will get the answers to these questions. We are interested in the quality of care delivered by you, and you alone sir."

"I have nothing to tell you, or your daughter, for that matter. You can talk to my lawyer!"

He stood up and went to the door. Please don't come back here again!" he said with venom, and showed Karl out of his office.

Returning to his desk, he placed a call to Foxworthy.

"James, that bitch Sharon has been talking to her father again, and he just left my office after a very unpleasant interview."

"Dr. Swenz, take it easy. I want you to tell our hospital attorney about the interview. I'll have him call you immediately."

Swenz slammed the receiver down and pounded his desk with his fist. "I'll kill her. She has interfered in my life for the last time. I hate her!" Rocking back on his chair, he began to rethink his position. He was in serious debt to his Vegas friends, and they had graciously extended his time for repayment of his gambling debts for two more weeks. He had to have $30,000 by then or else he was history. Both Michael Rome and David Malkin had promised to loan him the money to pay off the debt. They had already loaned large sums of cash to him over the past year for "debt consolidation" and were now very upset with him. They explained to him that he was jeopardizing everything they had all worked for and they weren't going to stand by and watch all their potential profits destroyed by him.

Of course, they were right. Their concern was that Swenz might do something stupid in order to gain money to pay off the debt and thereby expose himself needlessly to publicity, as well as to the law. They were completely dependent upon him to render the organ transplant patients their anti-rejection drug therapy since there was no one else who could be trusted with the Research Lab's secrets. Unknown to Swenz, he had been labeled as a loose cannon by the two CEOs, and they were desperate to see him out of their hair forever, but for that to happen, they had to first get FDA approval for KZ67.

The FDA had had the application for five months now and promised that it was at the top of the pile, but the filing process was still pending. Once the approval was granted for the use of KZ67, they wouldn't need Swenz, because any doctor would then be able to administer the drug with impunity. They would pay Swenz off per their agreement as soon as the cash flow was available from the worldwide sale of the cloned organs, the hepatitis D2 vaccine, and KZ67. This was all calculated to happen within a few months.

Swenz thought about Sharon and how she had notified the DOC to investigate TWMC through her father. He wasn't thinking rationally now, and decided he needed a drink.

~ 32 ~

THEY REALLY DO
COME IN THREES!

S haron finished up at the clinic and returned to her office. Subconsciously, she found herself rubbing her right
shoulder and suddenly became aware of a feeling of fullness
under her right arm. Quickly, she locked her office door and
took off her blouse, reaching into her right axilla with her left
hand. She palpated the area and became startled when she
thought she felt a mass.

"Oh my God!" she said aloud. Fear struck her heart and
she quickly dressed and placed a call to Michael. "Michael,
this is Sharon. I want to see you right away!"

"Of course, Sharon, come over to the office. I'll wait for
you."

She gathered her belongings and threw them into her
shoulder bag and headed for the elevator and the second
floor, which housed much of the medical services. She hastened her gait to Michael's office. He was at his desk doing
paperwork when she arrived.

"Sharon, come right in and have a seat," he said, pointing to a soft backed chair. "You look stressed out. What's the matter?"

"Michael, I want you to examine me right now. I think I feel something here," she said, pointing to her right armpit.

"Let's go to one of my clinic exam rooms." She followed him out the door and down the hall.

"Ruth," he said when they arrived, "please prepare Dr. Dell for a physical examination."

"Sure thing. Dr. Dell, in here please, and change into this lovely designer gown," she said with a grin as she tried to make light of the scene. Sharon changed into the examination gown and sat on the table awaiting Dr. Herbert. *Now I know what a patient goes through*, she thought to herself. *This is very stressful.*

"Let me take a history, Sharon," Michael said calmly.

"Have at it," replied Sharon.

At that point, he directed a barrage of medical questions to shed light on the issue at hand.

"Have you injured your hand in the past few weeks?"

"When I was fishing last week in Canada, I began to feel some pain in the right shoulder which I attributed to all the muscular exercise of reeling in heavy fish."

"Okay, was there any other injury?" he asked while taking her right hand into his. Sharon liked the feel of his hand on hers as he probed for areas of tenderness with his fingers. She was daydreaming and was awakened abruptly.

"Sharon, you have a small area of redness in the palm between the index and middle fingers. Did you injure yourself there?"

"Oh, how stupid of me. Yes, I got a fishhook in my hand, but there was no subsequent infection that I noticed."

"Place your right hand on my shoulder while I examine your axilla." He palpated the area and was surprised to find an enlarged lymph node, which felt harder than it should, as if it were reacting to inflammation from the hand. He then proceeded to do a more detailed examination assisted by his nurse, Ruth. When he completed the exam, he started to leave the room and turned to Sharon.

"Why don't you get dressed and meet me in my office, where we can talk alone?"

Sharon nodded and got off the table. She dressed and walked into his office, then sat down. "Well, what is your impression?"

"Sharon, uh … you do have a firm lymph node in the axillary chain. I want you to get a mammogram and ultrasound of the node tomorrow morning. Your history is negative, and it sounds to me like this is a reactive lymph node to a possible bacterial infection you sustained in the hand. The node is about three centimeters and firm. In view of the recent two cases that you sent to me, needless to say, I am not only amazed, but also very concerned."

"Me too."

"Look, tomorrow night we have a date. Why don't I pick you up and we can talk about the next step then, okay?"

"Fine, I'll be waiting for you. Here's my address." She handed him her professional card, and on the backside she had written her address. "See you then." She forced a smile. *Great*, she thought, *I am going on a first date with my doctor who has just seen me nude. Well that might be a plus, since he didn't offer an excuse to break the date.* She laughed at herself and strolled out to the elevators.

The next morning found Sharon in the Radiology Department, undergoing the testing procedures. She made a solemn promise to herself that she would always spend time explaining all testing procedures thoroughly to her patients so as to allay their fears and anxieties. It was very hard being a patient subjected to a variety of tests and feeling a loss of dignity as well. Here, they knew her, which made her feel additionally embarrassed. The testing was terminated shortly after noon, at which time Sharon went to the cafeteria. The room was very crowded, and as luck and would have it, she was forced to sit at a table for two with Barry Swenz. As she approached the table, he glared at her. "Do you mind if I sit here?" she asked.

Swenz was furious at the sight of her. "As a matter of fact, I do. I would appreciate being alone. I don't wish to speak with a traitor." Sharon gawked at Barry and couldn't believe what she had just heard him utter, and with such venom. Rather than responding, she walked away and eventually found a vacant chair at another table. Hurrying through her lunch, Sharon thought about the uncomfortable encounter with Barry a few short weeks before while waiting for the elevator. He had lost it then, and now he had repeated the performance.

She tried to piece it all together. Why was he so hateful toward her? After digesting the two encounters thoroughly, she came to the conclusion that Barry must think she was at the root of the DOC audit. But what about the previous meeting, when he'd professed indignation over the fact that his orders for surgery had been countermanded by her resident? The rationale offered by Barry just didn't ring true. Up to now, she hadn't given it much thought, but, thinking about it again raised other possibilities as to why Barry may have been upset. It was easy to connect the two outbursts now that today's event had occurred. *That has to be it! Barry is hostile at me because my father is working for the DOC, and he thinks that I must be responsible for him being here.* She left for home earlier than usual to get ready for her date with Michael.

It was 7:30 when the doorbell rang. "Who is it?" asked Karl. "It's Michael," replied the visitor, somewhat surprised to hear a male voice. Karl moved to the door and opened it."

"Hi, I'm Karl Dell, Sharon's father." There was a brisk handshake between the men, and Karl led Michael into the living room. "Please sit down. Sharon will only be a moment."

"I've heard a great deal about you from Sharon."

"No doubt all good things," said Karl with a grin.

"Yes sir, only the best, I assure you. How have you been since your liver transplant?"

"Just fine. I will be returning home to Auburn next week."

Sharon entered the room and walked toward Michael.

"Oh, Sharon," he said while standing up to greet her, "you are breathtaking." He nervously handed her a single ruby red rose.

"That was so thoughtful, Michael. Let me put this in a vase, I'll be right back."

Karl couldn't help but agree with the suitor. His daughter

was very beautiful indeed, he thought, and he was delighted to see her looking so exceptionally well. "You guys have fun," he said as he ushered them out the front door.

They drove away and headed west on the freeway. "Where are we going?" asked Sharon.

"Doctor, I am taking you to the finest restaurant in Los Angeles."

"Which one would that be?"

"Chinois, in Santa Monica."

"Got ya this time, Michael—that's not in Los Angeles!"

"You're correct. I was only checking to see if you were paying attention."

"Of course you were," she answered with compassion and understanding in her voice. They both laughed, and while they drove, Michael asked her to tell him about her recent fishing experience in Canada. She went into such detail that she hadn't concluded the story by the time they exited the Santa Monica Freeway at Fourth Street. They turned left and went to Pico Blvd, then turned right, and after two short blocks made a left on Main and then made a U turn pulling up in front of the restaurant. The valet took the car and they walked into the restaurant. Large picture windows allowed the diners to gaze out onto the sidewalk and be treated to the new generational fashion look. While they were waiting at the bar, they peered at the parade of spectacles on the street. They sat in silence, shaking their heads in amazement. "Is tonight Halloween?" Sharon asked with a suppressed laugh.

At that point they were shown to their table, where they could still observe the parade but could also witness the chef's at work creating culinary delights. The menu was large and the hors d'oeuvre were to die for. The entrée selection contained gustatory imaginations such as *Sizzling Catfish in Ginger and Ponzu Sauce, Shanghai Lobster in Spicy Ginger Curry Sauce and Crispy Spinach, Sauteed Louisiana Shrimp with Asparagus in warm Black Bean and Truffle Oil Sauce,* and *Mongolian Lamb Chops with Cilantro Vinaigrette and Wok Fried Vegetables.*

"This is really difficult, I can't decide what to order," said Michael.

"Why don't we just get a few different hors d'oeuvre rather than commit to a meal?" suggested Sharon.

"I like that idea. You are adventurous, aren't you Sharon?"

"When it comes to food, I am," she replied, taking a sip of her champagne cocktail." He took notice of the way she placed her lips on the wineglass and became intently interested in every movement she made. Desperately, he searched for body language indicating a *green light.* They each ordered two appetizers and split them. During dinner, Sharon asked Michael about himself. She concentrated on finding out what his tastes were in art, music and literature, not to mention sports, and was pleased to discover that his interests meshed with hers quite nicely. He loosened up after the second glass of Chardonnay, and by then, Sharon was feeling no pain as well. Michael took her hand on the table at one point in the conversation, and Sharon responded by gripping it tightly. Unconsciously, she slipped her foot next to his.

Michael read all of her signs and was very pleased, because he had strong feelings for her. He had been afraid to attempt any advances for fear she would reject him. He

looked into her soft dark eyes and saw a deeply compassion-
ate woman. He even thought he saw the mystical demeanor
of love radiating from the depths of her soul. Michael became entranced with Sharon's face and felt an intense longing
for her. This had never happened to him before, and he was
startled with this heartfelt desire. All his life, he had known
that he would recognize it when the right woman came along,
but now, he was uncertain. The more he thought about his
feelings, the more confused he became. He tried to put his
thoughts out of his mind, but to no avail.

The evening raced by, and, before they knew it, it was time
to leave. Michael hadn't had anything to drink for an hour
and felt safe enough to get behind the wheel. Sharon was de-
lightfully happy and fell asleep on his shoulder within minutes.
While she slept, Michael wrestled with himself for a plan. He
had blown the opportunity to discuss her radiology test results
at dinner. It just seemed so inappropriate then. He was more
interested in pursuing her on a social level, and the thought
of acting as her doctor was now very distasteful to him. He
finally came to grips with the situation and decided he would
speak with her by Monday, but in the meanwhile, he enjoyed
the scent of her perfume and the warmness of her head on
his shoulder. He placed his hand on her right thigh and gently
squeezed; he didn't want to awaken her. She responded with
a soft sigh, and then she awakened. Immediately, she grasped
his hand with both of hers and lightly kissed it.

"I like your hands," she said softly. "They are so strong
looking." Sharon stretched herself out on the seat with her
head next to his right thigh.

"I like your hands too. Your skin feels like velvet."

"Probably because of all the talc in the surgical gloves," she replied with a laugh. Michael looked into her face as she stared up at him. He was waiting for the light to change, and became mesmerized by her. "You know, you are very pretty even from this angle," he said with a laugh.

"And what exactly is that supposed to mean?" she asked, widening her eyes.

"It takes native beauty to look as good as you do from my line of sight. Your face is upside down and it is still beautiful."

"You are so sweet, and I thank you for the compliments; however, from my vantage point, I can't return them. Looking into two nostrils is not particularly flattering, you know."

Michael laughed and sped away at the change of the light. He pulled up in front of her condominium and parked the car. Without missing a beat, he grabbed her in his arms and kissed her for a long time. He felt her warm response and didn't want it to end. "I'd ask you in, Michael, but my dad is living with me a while longer."

"That's okay, it's very late anyway. May I call you tomorrow?"

"Please do, I'll be home all day." Sharon exited the car and Michael walked her to the front door. He looked into her dark eyes and kissed her gently on the lips. She acquiesced to his kiss and then stood with her arms around him and basked in her feelings of something very powerful for this man.

At two the next afternoon, Michael called her on the phone. "Can you meet me for coffee, Sharon?"

"Sure I can. Where do you want to meet?"

"What about Marie Callender's on Fifth Street?

"I'll be there in a half hour. See you then."

Michael hung up the phone and again rehearsed how he would present the facts to her.

Sharon entered the restaurant to find him sitting inside, awaiting her arrival. The hostess showed them to a booth, and they ordered coffee and relived the events of the night before. Then, at long last, he broached the subject.

"Sharon, I want to talk to you about your tests."

"You have the results already?"

"Yes, I called the radiologist yesterday and obtained them."

"Well, why didn't you tell me last night?" she asked with annoyance evident in her voice.

"I ... uh—I tried to, but you were having such a good time, I didn't want to talk about it then."

She realized he didn't have good news for her and felt a wave of nausea. "Michael, what is it?"

"The mammogram is normal, but the ultrasound is suspicious for malignancy," he said in a soft voice, looking away from her eyes.

"I can't believe it! I really thought the node enlargement was from the fishing hook in my hand. This whole thing is unreal."

"Sharon, I want to help you," he replied as he sought to find a place of comfort in her eyes. The eyes revealed fear, yet still held the look of confidence.

"What's next? A lymph node biopsy?"

"Yes, perhaps Monday afternoon. Would that be alright

with you?" He looked pleadingly at her and felt pain in his own heart.

"That's fine. Let's get it over with. By the way Michael, can you believe three women with the exact same presentation of solitary lymph node enlargement?"

"I'm having a lot of difficulty with that!" He reached over the table and took her hand in his. "Sharon, I have strong feelings for you, I think you probably know that."

"Michael, I'm perplexed. Everything is moving so fast. I feel the same way toward you, but this problem is draining me. I want you as my doctor, and I won't take no for an answer." She looked at him and smiled. She thought she saw approval in his eyes.

"I can't take care of you in an objective manner, Sharon, you know that. It would be much better if I transferred your clinical care to someone else."

"No way! You are stuck with me. I don't trust anyone else; the discussion is closed."

"Be reasonable! I have to be free to make decisions without an emotional bias."

"And what, kind sir, is that bias?"

"That, my dear lady, is the bias of a strong attachment."

Sharon became wide-eyed and grabbed his hands over the table. "Michael, please don't—"

Sensing her fear, along with his own embarrassment, he laughed and quickly sought to change the subject. "You will be fine! We'll beat this thing together."

Sharon felt a twinge of guilt about cutting him off so abruptly and wanted to explain. She sighed in relief when

Michael asked, "Why don't we sit in my car for a while before you leave?" "I was hoping you'd say that. I'd love to sit and ramble for a while, if you can take it."

They sat and he listened attentively while she expressed her fears, hopes and desires.

"I'm not certain of what I'm really feeling. You know how easily a grateful patient can mistake feelings. I won't even allow myself to meditate on any emotions. I'm too anxious and confused. I need to pass this hurdle in my life."

This catharsis continued for the better part of two hours, but to each of them, it only seemed like a few minutes. She felt refreshed when she concluded.

Monday afternoon, Sharon underwent a lymph node biopsy. She went home that night and told her father all about her condition. All of her surgery cases were canceled because of the postoperative pain and limitation of right upper extremity motion. The next morning, Michael came to her office and closed the door.

"Sharon, the biopsy is just like Ginny's and Gail's. It doesn't make sense!"

"I can't say I'm surprised. It was too much like their presentation not to be malignant."

"Sharon, I am going to culture the tumor cells. I already have them in culture from Ginny and Gail. The University Cancer Genetics Research Department will run some tests to see if we can get any clues."

"What do you mean, clues?"

"They will do a DNA analysis on each specimen to see if

any congenital abnormal gene is present. There is a lot that can be identified in this way."

"How long will this take?"

"About a week, they say."

"I guess I have no choices to make until then."

"Therapy will be dependent on what they find."

Sharon tried to stay busy with paperwork and catching up on the latest literature. She felt lucky to have Michael, as well as her father, but nevertheless, she was still anxious about the outcome. The days passed slowly and she spent them assuring her father that she was going to be all right, and each evening, she was infused with similar assurance by Michael.

~ 33 ~

THE DNA MESSAGE

It was just before noon eight days after her biopsy when Michael called. "Sharon, I must speak to you right away. Can I come to your office?"

"What is it?"

"I don't want to talk on the phone. I'll be right over. Okay?"

"I'll be here. Come over." In a few minutes, Michael walked into her office and closed the door behind him. "I have just received the results of the DNA analysis on all three cell cultures," said Michael in an excited voice.

"Well?" inquired Sharon as she started to pace in front of her desk.

"Sharon, please sit down, you won't believe this!"

"Okay, I'm sitting," she said with a somber expression.

"All three breast cancers have the exact same DNA. The cancer was derived from one source!"

Her mouth fell open in disbelief. "That means that it didn't develop from our own body cells!"

"Right, and what's more, it narrows the method of administration to each of you."

"Please explain."

"The only way three women could have received similar DNA would be through some sort of vector that had to be injected into each of you!"

"But—how? Where did it happen?"

"Think hard, Sharon. Have you received any injections of any kind in the last six months or so?" Sharon furrowed her brow and bit her lower lip. She stood up and began to pace again. Suddenly, she turned and clasped both her hands over her mouth in an attempt to stymie her spontaneous loud gasp. She ran to Michael and grabbed him by the arms and led him to a chair. "Michael, I received a hepatitis D2 immunization some six to eight weeks ago. Barry Swenz brought the vaccine to me and injected it into my right arm!"

"Oh my God!" He stood and wrapped his arms around her, pulling her close. She nestled her head on his chest for a blissful moment and sobbed softly. Abruptly, she pulled away. "Michael, I gave the immunization to Ginny and Gail later on the same day!"

"That explains it then. You injected them and all three of you came down with a cancerous axillary lymph node."

"Oh God, I gave them cancer and …" He took her by the hands and looked into her eyes. "No, you didn't, Sharon!"

She moved closer to him for comfort. "What are we going to do?"

"Did you immunize anyone else?"

"No."

"Do you remember how much was left in the vial?"

"There was only enough for maybe one more shot, but Gail and Ginny were the only ones around then, so I …"

"What Sharon, you did what?" She ran to her desk and opened the top right hand drawer and pulled out a glass vial. "I put it in my desk! Here it is, Michael."

Michael held the small vial up to the light and shook it. Rapidly, he read the label that confirmed it was hepatitis D2 Antigen and a broad smile came over his face. "What is it, Michael?"

"We can get answers now. I am going to take this to the University Genetics Lab myself. They will be able to perform a DNA analysis that should give us some answers." He started for the door and turned to Sharon. "I'll call you as soon as I know something."

"What about Swenz?"

"Don't say a word to him or anyone. Let's get all the goods first."

"But this is tantamount to attempted murder, Michael!"

"I agree, but we need to gather as much evidence as we can. Look, in addition to gathering evidence, we need to know the manner in which they produced the cancers, because it will dictate our treatment regimen."

"Okay, I'll leave it up to you. It's getting too deep for me now."

"Call you later." He literally ran from her office.

Michael entered University Hospital and took the elevator to the basement, where the genetics lab was located. Jack Kohl was a good friend of his ever since medical school days. Jack had elected to become a research scientist after completing a four-year program in genetics while at the National Institute of Health. He was a brilliant researcher and had contributed immensely to the area of cancer genetics. Sometimes, Michael felt his friend had the better job, since he didn't have to deal with the patient face-to-face.

"Hi Jack, how are you?"

"Doing great Michael. To what do I owe this visit?"

"It's a long story. Can we go somewhere private?"

"Certainly," said Jack, while opening the door to his private office. "So tell me about it.

"I sent you three separate cell cultures of breast cancer we obtained by lymph node biopsy. You reported that the DNA of all three was the same. Do you recall that?"

"Yes, I remarked that someone probably screwed up on labeling the cell cultures in order for all the DNA to be identical. I'll bet you are here to explain that labeling error and you brought the correct cell cultures with you. Right?"

"Wrong. But I did bring something else," he said as he withdrew a small vial from his jacket pocket. "There was no mistake in labeling the cultures. They came from three different women."

"Then there has to be an explanation, but I don't have one now."

"Precisely, and neither do I, but look what I've got here." He handed the small vial to Jack, who glanced at the label.

"It's labeled hepatitis D2 sntigen. What's this got to do with anything?"

"I don't believe it is antigen at all, and I'll bet my life it contains the answer."

"Please continue."

"This material was injected into each of the three women, and I'm betting there's a connection."

"I think you may be right. I can analyze for the presence of DNA. I'll be able to compare it to the three others and establish if they are all the same."

"Is it hard to do?"

"Not at all. We'll use the reflips method—restriction fragmentation length polymorphisms to determine if the DNA is of the same origin," he quickly added as he saw the look of bewilderment on his colleague's face. "After that, we'll use the PCR reaction to amplify the DNA strands, then run it through our computerized automatic DNA sequencer, which will identify the DNA and compare each sample to the solution in this bottle. If there is an oncogene in this bottle, we'll identify it and know if it was the cause of these cancers."

"Wonderful. How long will it take?"

"About twenty-four hours, if I start now."

"Okay, call me. I've got to run now."

"Will do, Jack. Good seeing you again."

"Jack held the small vial up to the light again and noticed that the label was smeared at the edge. He picked up his phone and dialed a number he knew by heart. His friend worked at the San Bernardino Sheriff's forensics department.

Back at TWMC, Michael related the nature of his discussions with Jack to Sharon. She felt good about everything she heard.

The following afternoon, Jack called Michael. "Michael, guess what we found?"

"I wouldn't know where to begin."

"We have a virus. It looks like an adenovirus. The viral genome is where the oncogene resides!"

"You mean the viral DNA has a human oncogene within it?"

"Exactly! We are in the process of growing the virus, and then we should be able to isolate and identify the oncogene even further."

"When will you know for sure?"

"In another thirty-six to forty-eight hours at the outside limit. I'll call you then."

Michael relayed the information to Sharon who was slightly disappointed that the testing hadn't been concluded yet.

It felt like two weeks rather than two days to Sharon before Michael called her with the results of the genetic testing.

"The results are conclusive, Sharon. The DNA testing shows that the adenovirus contained an oncogene for breast cancer, and it's the same DNA that's in the actual cancer."

"That means that the virus-incorporated DNA oncogene came from someone else's breast cancer cells."

"That's really sick, isn't it?"

"Yes, it is. What do we do now?"

"Doctor Kohl at the University Genetics Lab has been working on cancer suppression gene therapy to cure cancer. I have asked Jack to test the cancer for its response to the cancer suppressor gene p53, which codes for p53 protein. This protein leads the abnormal cancer cells to their own death by apoptosis. He can add this gene to an adenovirus and deliver it into the cancer cell by injection. When an adenovirus enters a normal cell, p53 protein responds by shutting down the host cells manufacture of its own DNA. This then prevents further replication by the virus. This is a drawback, because the viruses will not multiply. We want as many viruses as we can get to enter the cancer cells. He figured out a way to disable the protein from suppressing viral multiplication. The p53 gene was altered so the virus will only grow in cells that lack normal p53, like the cancer cell. These modified viruses grow rapidly in cancer cells and produce daughter viruses, which are also armed with the same ability to kill these cells by instructing the cancer cell to die."

"When will we know?" "It may take a few weeks to get the answer, but if the cells respond, all we need to do is inject the three of you with another adenovirus to get a cure."

"I pray you are right. This waiting is starting to get to me."

-34-

TIME TO ACT

Karl Dell was engrossed in discussion with his boss, Dr. John Higgins. "Tell me again what Swenz said to you," asked John in amazement.

"I asked him why he was the only doctor who was following the post-transplant patients. I pointed out to him that the usual and customary manner dictates treatment of a patient be provided by the appropriate specialist and not an orthopedist."

"His answer?"

"Since all that is required is adjustment of drug dosage for any rejection process, any doctor trained in the use of the anti-rejection drugs can do it."

"How did you respond?"

"I informed him that the Medical Board of California does not hold that view. He responded that all doctors should care for the entire patient and not only their narrow specialty area."

"Well, he must have backed off somewhat, didn't he?"

"Not one iota! After I got nowhere, I then reminded him

about the residence training programs, which train doctors to be competent in specialty areas. In a weak moment, he told me that he had agreed to follow the postoperative transplant patients because there was no one else available to provide that service. I asked him who he had agreed to do that for, and he screamed at me and told me it was none of my business."

"And that was it?"

"No, he really lost control then. He accused my daughter, who works at TWMC, of putting me up to the audit and then threw me out of his office."

"Okay, I've got the picture now. Stay here for a moment while I place a few calls." He began to dial the telephone number of the Medical Board of California. His longtime friend, Dr. William Caldarone, was Chief of the Enforcement Section, which was charged with the responsibility of physician oversight. They were the state agency that watched over all medical practitioners and, where applicable, investigated and prosecuted those who violated the law.

"Hello Bill, this is John Higgins at the DOC."

"Yes, John, how can I help you?"

"I need some assistance in a pressing matter the DOC is investigating."

"I'll try to lend a hand."

"The DOC has done an extensive medical audit at TWMC and uncovered severe irregularities in a physician's practice pattern. He is an orthopedist who is the treating doctor for all postoperative transplant patients operated on at TWMC. These are only patients who belong to World Health Care

HMO. His position is that he is able to do this because managing the anti-rejection drugs can be done by anyone trained in that area and he denies that it requires a specialist to do so. He even cares for the pediatric cases."

"That is highly irregular behavior. A pediatrician trained in the area of the organ replacement would be the proper one to care for the patient."

"You mean a gastroenterologist for a liver transplant and a nephrologist for a kidney?" "That would be appropriate for adults, but for kids, they would have to be pediatric G.I. or renal specialists."

"I am in agreement with that. Will you investigate this, or shall we go directly to the attorney general's office with it?"

"Why don't you file a complaint with the board, and then we will start an immediate investigation? If you fax me the complaint, I'll authorize our San Bernardino investigators to get right on it."

"I guess we have to wait until you complete your investigation before anything can be done to stop this practice."

"That's right, but you can shorten the process for us drastically if you'll copy all the information you have collected and your department's findings on the matter."

"It's on the way, Bill, and thanks for the help."

"By the way, who is the orthopedist?"

"Doctor Barry Swenz."

"I'll check our computer files for anything negative. Talk to you later."

– 35 –

WHEN ERRORS ARE MADE

B arry Swenz entered his weekly clinic, where he was in charge of the follow-up care of all postoperative transplant patients. His job was to decide the dosage of KZ67 required to stave off any rejection process. He was agitated over the recent visit by Karl Dell, but he projected all his venom onto Sharon, his colleague. She was the cause of all his pain and anxiety, and he was basking in joy over the hospital gossip that Sharon had metastatic breast cancer. Often, he would try to calculate how quick the cancer would kill her. With her gone, there would be no one to testify against him if anything happened as a result of the DOC investigation. He had his life to live, and with the threat of losing his medical license, there wouldn't be much left to it. The gambling debts were always there and had to be satisfied, but as soon as he was paid by Rome and Malkin, he would pay off his debts and retire in another country. His mind was continually preoccupied with these thoughts and not on the task at hand, which was rendering care to his patients.

Sandra Firestone was forty-four years old and a mother of two. She had undergone a liver transplant a little over a year ago at TWMC and was being followed in Swenz's clinic. Over the past two months, there had been a slow upward creeping of her bilirubin and liver enzyme levels. Despite the insidious nature of the blood levels and her complaining to Doctor Swenz about fatigue, loss of appetite, and diffuse severe joint pains, Swenz did nothing, and indeed today she was in pain as well.

"How are you today, Sandra?" asked Swenz matter of factly. He was still ruminating about his personal dilemma as he looked through his patient's medical chart.

"My pain is worse, Doctor," she replied in a whimper. She had tears in her eyes as she spoke, but they went unnoticed. Swenz entered a note into the chart, *Joint pains continue and liver function tests getting worse.*

"You know, your lab tests are abnormal, which means you are having an acute rejection process, so I am going to increase the KZ67 dose and add a small amount of steroids."

"How long will it take before I feel better?"

"Hopefully within a week or so," he answered spontaneously without any evidence of really caring. He checked her record to see what the diagnosis was that led to the failure of her own liver more than a year ago. Finding the discharge summary for the transplant hospitalization, he noticed the diagnosis of "hepatitis" and was satisfied.

"What about the pain here?" she replied, pointing to her left upper abdomen. "Don't you want to examine me?"

"That's to be expected. I'll see what the blood tests show."

Sandra got up to leave, aided by the nurse, while Swenz continued to see the rest of the patients who were waiting patiently for him.

Three days later, Doctor Swenz received a call from Sandra Firestone complaining of severe weakness. Unable to get out of bed, she had vomited blood earlier that morning. "You'd better come into the ER and be seen now, Sandra. I'll call the ambulance to pick you up." He hung up the phone. "Damn it!"

Shortly thereafter, the ER physician called Swenz to inform him that his patient had just arrived in the ER DOA. Swenz sighed and shook his head. He had done his job. It wasn't his fault that she'd died from a rejection of the donor liver. These things did happen to these patients. He went on about his work not caring the least bit about the death of his patient and the somber fact that two children were now without their mother.

It didn't take but a few weeks for Mr. Firestone to engage the services of the noted malpractice attorney, Jason Nichols. A few weeks later, Doctor Swenz became acutely aware of Mr. Firestone's actions.

"Are you Doctor Swenz?" asked the small man, trying to keep up with Swenz's pace.

"Yes, I am," answered Swenz, annoyed at the interruption. He harbored general dislike for anyone who barged in on his privacy, but more so when it happened to him at TWMC.

"This is for you." He handed him some papers, then

walked away. Swenz peered at the heading on the first page: *You have been sued!*

Quickly, he shoved the papers in his pocket, and when he got to his office, he withdrew them again as he sat at his desk. He was being sued for wrongful death by Mr. Firestone, and the complaint alleged he had misdiagnosed and mistreated Sandra, which had caused her death. He also noticed that TWMC was named as a defendant in the case. His emotions were a combined hatred, fear, and paranoia. He lurched at the phone on his desk and sent it sliding across his desk while he held the handset to his ear. Mumbling to himself aloud, he walked around the desk to retrieve the rest of the telephone from the floor. "Put Foxworthy on now," he ordered.

"Is this Doctor Swenz?" his secretary inquired in a straightforward manner.

"Yes, and I don't have all damn day," he gruffly replied.

"Please hold." The line went dead for a few seconds.

"James Foxworthy here," came the saccharin sweet voice that immensely irritated Swenz.

"Have you been served yet?" inquired Swenz sarcastically.

"On the Firestone case, yes. I have already sent it over to the attorney."

"What are you going to do for me with regard to it it?"

"What do you mean?"

"I mean that I let my malpractice insurance lapse last year because I couldn't afford the fifty-thousand-dollar premium." He knew he was perpetrating a lie as he recalled the circumstances surrounding the payment. He had the money set aside for the premium; however, he also had been visited by his friends from Las Vegas. It was one of those periods in his life that were occurring very frequently now, forcing him to settle his gambling debts. There was no room for negotiations with those people, and he'd opted to forego payment of the medical malpractice premium, but not without promising himself he would call the company and try to get an extension on his coverage. The company had agreed to accept a five-thousand-dollar payment and place his account on a monthly payout. No matter—Swenz had never found the five thousand dollars available to make the monthly payments, and the malpractice policy had lapsed a month later. But he remembered that he had promised himself that he would restore the insurance just as soon as he had the funds. Needless to say, that day never came. Every available dollar Swenz received went to pay off his continuing casino debts.

"Doctor Swenz, you know very well that malpractice insurance is every doctor's personal responsibility and is not the hospital's." "Now you listen and listen real well! I have stuck my neck out for your lousy hospital as well as Genome, Bently, and World Health Care for years. All of you better get together and decide how you are going to cover my legal fees, because I don't have the funds for it. If you give me any crap about it, I just might reveal the whole plan to the authorities, so you make the decision. Let me know by tonight what you decide!"

"I will talk to the others and get back to you later on today." Foxworthy sat behind his desk and rubbed his head. He felt one of those blockbuster headaches coming on and knew the rest of his day was now ruined.

The medical board acted quickly to gather information about Doctor Swenz, as well as TWMC. Two investigators were assigned to the task at hand. When they had completed their information search, they discussed the findings with Doctor Bernard Gannon, the medical consultant to the San Bernardino district. He tried to get Swenz to come to his office for an interview, but his attempt was in vain. The law did not require a physician to appear for such an interview, but it certainly created a negative impression with the board if the party refused. It was not a legal process at all, but was only for the purpose of posing questions to issues uncovered by the investigators in the hope that some of the answers would dispel further need to investigate or even prosecute. Gannon was left no choice but to meet with the assistant attorney general and request that he file a petition with the court immediately for an Interim Suspension Order immediately against Doctor Swenz, as well as TWMC.

Attorney General David Braun walked into Doctor Gannon's office. "Doctor Gannon, I am David Braun with the AG's office."

"Please sit down and I'll get right to the point. We have investigated circumstances surrounding questionable practices of Doctor Barry Swenz, an Orthopedist, who practices exclusively at TWMC. Our investigators have found that he is practicing in areas in which he is not qualified or trained." He then related in detail all the information supplied by the DOC in their medical audits. "Our investigators have also been told by nurses and others at TWMC that Swenz has been acting very odd for some time now. The charts reveal that he is administering an anti-rejection drug called KZ67, which looks like a research protocol, without patient consent, and there is no evidence of the drug having been approved by the FDA. We have also found that he visits Las Vegas almost every weekend and the rumors are he has a gambling addiction. One of my investigators went to Las Vegas and confirmed these rumors and also that he loses a great deal of money on his weekend visits."

"Was he able to find out the amount he loses?"

"He was told it wasn't unusual for him to lose ten thousand dollars at a clip."

"That might be the driving force here."

"What do you mean?"

"Well, Swenz has gotten himself in a very bad financial situation, which may be why he is committing himself to jeopardy on the many fronts you have told me about. Perhaps his motive is the gambling debt."

"I never gave that a thought. It doesn't excuse him, but it explains the reason, maybe."

"I believe there is enough here to file a petition with the court for an ISO hearing. As you know an Interim Suspension Order will be heard by an administrative law judge. I will need you to help me obtain declarations from medical experts who will testify that Swenz's behavior represents an extreme deviation from the standard medical practice and places his patients at extreme risk. As far as TWMC is concerned, I can enlist Doctor Karl Dell's testimony and hopefully shut down their transplantation service temporarily. It would be great if we had one of their own doctors testify for us."

"Let me look into that for you."

"Fine then, I'll let you know when the hearing date is set." Gannon accompanied the AG to the door. "Dianne, please get me the CEO at TWMC."

"Right away, sir." After a brief pause, she spoke again. "Mr. Foxworthy on line two, Doctor."

"Mr. Foxworthy, this is Doctor Bernard Gannon of the Medical Board Enforcement Division in San Bernardino. I am the medical consultant assigned to this office and I would like to speak with you for a moment about an issue relating to your facility."

"Certainly Doctor, how may I help you?"

"A complaint has been filed against one of your doctors and your hospital by the DOC. We have thoroughly investigated the issue and have asked the Attorney General's Office to file a petition with the court for an Interim Suspension Order, which would effectively stop your hospital from performing further transplantation surgeries and stop the physician from practicing immediately."

Foxworthy began to sweat profusely. The transplant program was responsible for an essential part of his hospital's profit, not to mention the effect it would have on World Health Care's stock once the news broke. Industries and employers would easily bail out of World in favor of a competing HMO. This was just not the right time for this to happen. The joint venture partners certainly would all suffer if any severe losses were sustained by any one of the partners. That fact had been agreed to in the very beginning, over four years ago. No one would receive any of the profits until the company's losses were made whole first, and Lord knew that would eat up all the profits available for distribution. He swallowed hard against the rising lump in his throat and found it hard to speak with his mouth so dry. "Who, may I ask, is the doctor?" He was already quite sure of the answer he was about to hear, but he had to play the part of a surprised and shocked CEO.

"Doctor Barry Swenz."

There it was. First a civil lawsuit for wrongful death, and now this by the medical board. "How is the hospital implicated, sir?"

"We have evidence that would lead us to believe there have been numerous acts within the hospital that have gone unchecked and that are dangerous to the well-being of patient care. I would like to interview one of the transplant surgeons myself. Who would you suggest I speak with?"

Foxworthy was quick to reply. "Doctor Sharon Dell would be the one." He was certain she would be neutral with regard to any of the hospital's liability issues, and her surgical outcomes were exemplary, which should impress that snoop Gannon.

"Thank you Mr. Foxworthy, I'll call her," he said.

Foxworthy hung up, took a big breath and then personally called all the members of the joint venture and insisted that they meet to discuss this round of events. He was also thinking about the money he would shortly receive from the partnership while the pain in his head grew steadily worse as he pondered the ominous possibilities.

The meeting was called to order by Michael Rome. The

room was perceptive with anxiety and fear communicated among the partners through glances. David Malkin sat next to the powerful Seymour Kramer, while James Foxworthy sat across the long sleek conference table from the others. Foxworthy liked to be at a vantage point whenever they met. In this manner, he was able to keep the faces of the others in sight, and in so doing, felt comfortable in interpreting their expressions. As was his custom, he sided with the most powerful of the lot, which had always kept him on the right side of the movers and shakers. He placed the legal pad in front of him and began to make notes as he looked at each man at the table and attempted to read their innermost thoughts before beginning his presentation to the group.

"Thank you all for coming here on such short notice, but I had no choice in calling this meeting, as I am certain you will all agree. I received a telephone call from the Medical Board of California this morning which concerned me greatly. They are filing a petition with the court to stop TWMC from performing any more transplants, and are also asking the court to suspend Doctor Swenz's practice of medicine."

"What on earth for," asked Malkin with extreme concern, as evidenced by his frown.

"Swenz is being accused of improper practice because he delivers the postoperative care to all the transplant patients and they don't think he has the expertise and training to do so. TWMC is accused of allowing non-FDA-approved drug testing on these patients and failure to inform the patients that these were research drugs not yet approved for clinical use."

"My God, they're sure to track this to us," said Rome in a panic.

"And if that happens, we are sure to be exposed as well!" blurted Malkin.

"We have the most to lose immediately if this hits the press," said Kramer. "All the large companies who have their health plans with us will bail out. Our stockholders will all beat a path to their brokers and sell. Our stock will plummet!"

"Gentlemen, what about us?" asked Foxworthy. "We also have a great deal to lose since transplant surgery is a large contributor to our financial success. Remember we depend heavily upon World Health for their volume of transplants as well as their other business. The medical marketplace for hospital patients is extremely competitive now. Why, it's possible we might face financial ruin as well!"

"Please, everyone, calm yourselves for a moment and let's examine the problem in more detail," suggested Rome. "Swenz is the major problem here. His gambling will no doubt be uncovered. Perhaps we can unload the entire problem on him. We have advanced him funds on a number of occasions because of his huge debts. He is a loser, and I, for one, would like to use him to our benefit. We have enough backup data to support our contention that we filed in a timely manner with the FDA for approval of organ cloning for transplantation. If you recall, we gathered all the data and changed the dates to appear as if the studies were all current. Swenz was the one who told the Pharmacy and Therapeutics Committee that KZ67 had FDA approval. None of us ever said that! Make sure that Barotta has copies of the minutes of that meeting. Foxworthy, you have assured me that all the hospital records will be in sync with our dates, correct?"

"We have done that. All records reflect the proper dates to back up your reporting data." Rome interrupted. "The FDA will never go to the patient for a confirmation of the date of surgery. They just don't do that type of investigating. They are only interested with the trial data that we report, so the remaining issues are as follows: Swenz is not qualified to administer anti-rejection drug treatment in all patients. Our position will be that we engaged him to be the director of the program and oversee the other doctors who were actually doing the work but he duped us. He billed us for all the work but it was his responsibility to hire the appropriate specialists and pay them. We contracted with him and he was to subcontract to the others. It just so happens that we have his signature on an agreement which states this in small print." He laughed aloud and looked around the table for confirmation. He saw smirks from everyone and knew he had hit on the solution.

"This should exonerate all of us on this point. Your position will be," he continued, looking directly at Foxworthy, "that the KZ67 was in a clinical research protocol, which required the patients' knowledge and acceptance of this treatment and, no doubt, your Pharmacy and Therapeutics Committee minutes will reveal KZ67 was approved for clinical research by the medical staff at the time we began to use it here at TWMC. I am certain those minutes would also reflect Doctor Swenz's position as director of the clinical research trials and that he was charged with the responsibility of securing the informed consent of every patient in which the drug was used."

"As I recall," said Foxworthy, "the informed consent for organ transplantation also has a clause regarding the use of KZ67 within it."

"That may also be helpful to you."

"I have taken the liberty of asking Andrew Barotta, hospital counsel, to be here to answer questions about the legal procedures. He is outside now waiting. Shall we invite him in?"

"Yes, I think we would all feel better hearing from him," answered Kramer.

Foxworthy walked to the door and, in a moment, returned with Barotta. "This is our hospital counsel gentlemen, Andrew Barotta."

Andrew greeted each of the men with a handshake and then sat down next to Foxworthy and waited to be recognized.

"Mr. Barotta, what can you tell us about the impending legal proceedings?" asked Malkin.

"Let me begin by explaining how things will proceed. I have been in discussion with the attorney general's office about the issues. They will file a petition with the court tomorrow on behalf of the medical board requesting the court grant an Interim Suspension Order. This will be heard by an administrative law judge who will decide whether the facts submitted warrant the extreme action. The board will present expert medical witnesses and submit medical declarations regarding the necessity of the order to safeguard the health and safety of the public. We may also present witnesses on our behalf, but not until the second hearing. That will be in fifteen days, at which time the court will hear further evidence. The court then may dismiss the complaint or continue the ISO for another thirty days, at which time a full hearing on the merits of the case will be heard and an adjudication will be made by the court."

"Who will testify for us tomorrow?" asked Foxworthy.

"I will put Doctor Dell on the stand to testify as to the necessity of continuing the transplant surgery. At such short notice, I'm not certain who else I will use tomorrow."

"Will you also be representing Swenz?"

"Yes, I think it would be appropriate to do so. If you gentlemen don't require my presence any more, I have a lot of preparation to do this evening."

"Call us after the hearing. What time is it set for?" asked Rome.

"One p.m., and James, I think you should be there with us."

"Fine, I'll be there. I think I'll check on the medical staff minutes we discussed earlier, gentlemen, so if no one has an objection, I suggest the meeting be adjourned."

That evening, Andrew Barotta discussed the case and the salient hospital issues with Sharon, who agreed to testify in court.

▲ ▲ ▲

At 1 p.m., Barotta entered the courtroom along with Doctor Dell, Swenz, and James Foxworthy. Assistant Attorney General David Braun spread his evidence on the table before him. His witnesses were Bernard Gannon, M.D., who

represented the Medical Board of California, and Karl
Dell, M.D., representing the Department of Corporations of
the State of California.

Judge Adam Kelly was on the bench reviewing the documents previously submitted by the State. "Mr. Braun, you
may begin."

"Your Honor, the State is petitioning the court for an
ISO against TWMC and Doctor Barry Swenz on the basis
that each one has contributed an extreme departure from the
standard of practice in the specific areas of transplantation
surgery and in the medical follow-up of the patients after surgery. In the case of TWMC, we shall show that the hospital
has failed to meet the standards by not following both state
and federal rules. The violations are as follows:

Failure to obtain informed consent for the use of a non-
FDA-approved drug. Failure to certify the competency of
Doctor Swenz for practicing medicine in areas in which he is
not sufficiently trained, and allowing the use of a non-FDA
approved drug in the hospital. Doctor Swenz is charged with
extreme departure from the standard of practice in this state
with regard to his use of the drug KZ67. He is also charged
with the use of a non-FDA-approved drug and failure to obtain specific informed consent for a research protocol. The
final charge is that his behavior represents a severe departure from standard and the suspicion that he is an impaired
physician."

"Call your first witness, please."

"Doctor Karl Dell."

"Please raise your right hand." He was sworn in and took

his seat on the stand. "Please tell us what your investigation uncovered that led to the medical board's intervention."

"I was instructed to audit TWMC to ascertain the quality of care being given to patients after they received their transplant surgery. I found many irregularities in that area and filed a complaint with the medical board." Karl described some of the irregularities, as well as his meeting with Swenz. "The DOC feels that in view of the irregularities we uncovered, the transplant program should be halted." It grieved him to make that statement, because he knew how it would hurt Sharon. Life was strange, wasn't it? Here he was trying to stop a program in which his daughter's life was so entrenched! He knew what he had to say might close the program she had worked so hard to build. She had said that she understood what he had to do and to her credit, he thought, she had learned strong morals and ethics, and was now demonstrating those years of teaching with immense strength.

When he concluded his testimony, Doctor Gannon was sworn in and confirmed Karl's findings. In addition he submitted affidavits from medical experts who also agreed with their position on the issues.

Mr. Barotta asked for a private meeting with the DA. He showed him the minutes of the Pharmacy and Therapeutics medical staff committee minutes where Doctor Swenz's statement to the committee was that the drug KZ67 was an FDA-approved drug for research. The committee minutes also reflected the fact that Swenz had been appointed as the Director of Clinical Research by both TWMC, as well as The Research Laboratories, and his duties were listed in the contract agreement enclosed as part of the minutes. The DA read the contract and saw that Swenz was charged with the supervision of the clinical research, but he was also to employ other physician specialists as the program demanded. Furthermore, he was also made responsible through the signed contract to obtain informed consent of all patients where KZ67 was administered. The DA smiled when he was shown the documents and rapidly agreed to dismiss TWMC with prejudice from the action.

"TWMC calls Doctor Sharon Dell to the stand." Sharon stood and walked to the stand and sat down, allowing her gaze to sweep the room. She smiled at her father, who was busy looking at the scattered documents in front of him on the table. He returned her gaze and smiled back. Braun walked to the front of the table and waited while the clerk administered the oath to Sharon.

"Your Honor, the State has agreed to stipulate to Doctor Dell's expert witness qualifications."

"Is that so, Mr. Braun?" asked Judge Kelly, peering over his spectacles.

"Yes, Your Honor, we will so stipulate."

"Proceed, Mr. Barotta, but first, is there a relationship between the two Doctor Dells?"

"Yes your honor, they are father and daughter."

"Thank you for explaining that to me. I was a bit surprised, but now I am surprised even further." The court was silent for what felt like an hour and finally Barotta stood up.

"Doctor Dell, how long have you been employed by TWMC?"

"I believe it will be about two years next month."

"Please tell the court what you do at TWMC."

"I am a transplant surgeon and assistant department chairperson. My job is to see that the transplant program functions at the highest level, and I'm also responsible for the training program within my department. About fifty percent of my time is spent in surgery performing transplant surgery. Since the hepatitis epidemic six months ago, I have had to spend eighty percent of my time performing surgery."

"Now Doctor, did you speak with Doctor Bernard Gannon of the medical board?"

"Yes I did."

"What did you tell him?"

"I told him that TWMC is the only regional hospital that can do transplants and, if we are precluded from operating, many people will die. I also told him that Doctor Swenz had been acting strange for some months now and that he had injected a substance into my arm that caused me to develop breast cancer." She stared at Swenz, who was fuming. His face was beet red and he fidgeted nervously in his chair.

"Please be more specific with regard to the hospital's position in the community for the transplant surgery."

"TWMC is the tertiary referral for organ transplantation surgery. We perform more than seventy-five percent of the transplants done from Sacramento to San Diego. We already have a waiting list, as well as scheduled patients who are in desperate need for transplants. Many will die if we cannot do the surgeries." "Now, Doctor, please elaborate on the injection Doctor Swenz gave you and your allegation that it caused cancer." Sharon reiterated her story and brought the court up to date on the research done at University Hospital. When she concluded, the room was extremely silent. She was then asked to recall the abnormal behavior of Barry Swenz to the court. She looked at her father when she concluded her testimony. She felt remorseful now that Karl had heard her testimony, because she had never told him of the cancer. He was desperately trying to hide the tears in his eyes, but without success. Their testimony was convincing to the court. The recess lasted twenty minutes, and during this time, Barotta and Assistant AG Braun struck a deal. The judge resumed the hearing and asked Mr. Braun to begin his defense. "Your Honor, may we approach the bench?"

"Alright." He motioned to the court recorder to come to the bench also. Just then, Swenz turned to Foxworthy, "You bastards are selling me down the river, aren't you?" He then made an attempt to grab Foxworthy's jacket but missed as the other man withdrew quickly from reach. Swenz's voice became loud and threatening, which prompted the judge to look over the bench. "Order in the court!" He slammed the gavel down hard. "Doctor, I will ask you to leave if I hear another outburst." Swenz stared at Foxworthy with hate and sat back in his seat.

"Your Honor," said the Assistant AG, "the State has reached a compromise at this point with one of the defendants."

"What is it?"

"The State would be willing to withdraw its ISO petition request against TWMC at this point and allow you to rule on the evidence against Doctor Swenz only. We have obtained certain guarantees that will be put into action at TWMC to safeguard the patients."

"Is that alright with you, Mr. Barotta?"

"Yes your Honor, it is." They all returned to their places and the judge cleared his throat.

"This is on the record. The State has withdrawn its petition against TWMC only. It is the finding of this court that certain guarantees by TWMC for a corrective action plan for the safeguard of the patients shall be instituted immediately. They shall include, but are not limited to, providing appropriate medical specialists to render the care appropriate to all patients who are or who will be placed on the drug KZ67. Furthermore, those plans shall be submitted within forty-eight hours to the medical board and the DOC for their joint approval. Upon approval, TWMC may continue to provide transplant surgery without interruption.

"In the matter of Doctor Barry Swenz, the court finds more than enough evidence to grant the State's petition for an ISO. Court will resume a second hearing on this matter in fifteen days. The clerk will notify you tomorrow of the time. Court adjourned." The judge walked from the bench and left the courtroom, unaware that Swenz was approaching Barotta.

"So I am the fall guy, right Barotta?" screamed Swenz as he shoved the attorney with both his hands. Barotta fell backward and then fell on one knee.

"Doctor Swenz, you had better quit while you are ahead!" Braun caught the events and rushed over to restrain Swenz, who was now screaming at the top of his voice. "I'll get all of you. Wait and see. TWMC will go down big time when I finish with them!"

He ran from the courtroom.

"It's a good thing this hearing was here and not in Superior Court where there are bailiffs present. Swenz might have been put in jail for a while after an outburst like that," said Braun. Everyone was nerve-racked as they gathered their belongings and walked to the street. Sharon walked with her father and tried to make peace, through abundant explanations, over her failure to tell him about her medical problem. He understood her reasons but nevertheless was still in a state of disbelief over the entire issue. "It's bad enough that father and daughter end up on as witnesses on different sides of the case, but I just feel hurt you didn't confide in me about your health problems." "Dad, I didn't want you to worry about me—you have enough to worry about with your own health, never mind having to be concerned with mine." She gave him a peck on the cheek.

-36-

CHANGING THE CODE

It was shortly before noon when Michael placed the call to Sharon.

"Sharon, I just got off the phone with Doctor Kohl at the University Lab, and I've got great news!" he shouted into the telephone.

"Tell me!"

"He has been able to alter the p53 gene. Remember what I told you? The p53 gene codes for a protein that instructs a cell with abnormal DNA to kill itself, and those are the cancer cells. The virus has been engineered so that it will only reproduce in these cancer cells. As the virus invades the cancer cell, the p53 protein will cause the cell to die."

"Is he sure it will work one hundred percent?"

"He is certain that it will, and he has prepared the genetically engineered adenovirus for immediate use on all three of you."

"When can you get it over here?"

"I told him that I would pick it up later today."

"Great Michael, I'll wait in my office for you, and in the meanwhile, I'll notify the others of the good news."

"See you later." Sharon felt the warmth spreading over her. She was exhilarated. For the first time in many weeks, she felt the ominous cloud over her life lifting, and she could see and feel the ray of sunshine. Subconsciously, she placed her hand in her axilla and felt the hard mass, but this time, she didn't feel despair.

Michael showed up on time, as promised, and withdrew the small bottle of clear fluid from his pocket. He pulled up one cc into the syringe and injected it into her right shoulder. "The viruses will find their way to the lymph nodes just like before, but now they will seek and destroy all the cancer cells."

"Let's go to the clinic and administer the virus to Ginny and Gail."

When they got there, Michael rapidly explained the action of the virus to both, who agreed to take the injection. Afterward, he explained to them that the wrong drug had been given to Sharon by Doctor Swenz and there was an investigation going on concerning the "error." Sharon had pleaded with Michael not to disclose the truth about Swenz yet because of the distrust it would cause within the hospital. "I want to examine each of you every week to keep tabs on the effect of this virus." They all agreed to return weekly to his office for their appointments.

"Come back to my office with me," said Sharon. Michael followed her into the elevator and they walked to the office, where they were alone at this late hour. Sharon sat next to him.

"Michael, no matter what happens, I want you to know that I care for you." Sharon felt compelled to let him know her feelings for him. "I can almost reach my feelings now that I know I have a real chance of a cure. Before today, I didn't care about anything really. It was impossible for me to imagine anything on a long-term basis until now. I am so grateful to you." They sat together for an hour and talked about the future and enjoyed each other's company. Finally, she said she had to go home and tell her father. Michael was content as he walked her to the door, then departed himself.

~ 37 ~

THE DEPOSITION

The next two weeks flew by. Sharon, Gail and Ginny all had reductions in the size of their lymph nodes, which was interpreted by Doctor Michael Herbert as an excellent response to the injection of the genetically engineered p53 gene.

In front of Judge Adam Kelly, the State presented witnesses to convince him to continue the ISO on Doctor Barry Swenz, and to no one's surprise, the ISO was not lifted. The next hearing on the merits of the accusation was scheduled for thirty days. Swenz never came to the second hearing and had not yet hired his own attorney to defend him. It just so happened that he was so deeply involved in the wrongful death suit brought by Mr. Firestone on behalf of his deceased wife that he failed to remember the date of the second ISO hearing. The deposition was taken in the offices of Mr. Jason Nichols, attorney for the plaintiff, while Swenz was represented by Mr. Bert Rawley.

"Have you ever had your deposition taken before, Doctor?" asked Nichols.

"No."

"A deposition is the same as testifying on the stand in court. It carries the same weight. You have been given an oath that is the same oath given in a court of law. Even though we are in the relaxed setting of an office, I must caution you to tell the truth as though you were in front of a judge and jury. Failure to do so carries with it the penalty of perjury. I am entitled to ask you questions, and if you don't understand them, please ask me to repeat or rephrase them. When you answer, you are not to guess, but you are required to give me your best estimate. Please wait until I have finished the question so your complete answer can be taken down by the court reporter. We don't want her to miss anything due to both of us speaking at the same time. When the deposition is transcribed, you will have a chance to review it in detail and make any additions, deletions or corrections, but if you do make any changes, I will be able to comment upon them at the time of trial. Now, is there any reason you cannot testify here today?"

"What do you mean?"

"Well, are you taking any medications yourself that might impair your ability to think properly?"

"No."

"Are you ill in any way today?"

"No, I am not."

"Alright then, Doctor—please state your whole name and date of birth for the record."

"Barry Swenz. September 10, 1957."

"Would you describe your educational background?"

"Mr. Nichols," interrupted Rawley, "I have taken the liberty of preparing Doctor Swenz's curriculum vitae, which might avoid the necessity of going through his history." He handed the document to Nichols who sat back in his chair and studied the three pages. "I will accept this, Mr. Rawley, and will instruct the reporter to mark this defendant's 'A'." He then handed the document to Swenz. "Is this your current CV, Doctor?"

"Yes it is."

"Doctor Swenz, how did you come to know Mrs. Sandra Firestone?"

"She was a patient that I cared for since her liver transplant surgery."

"Where did you render that care?"

"At TWMC, in my transplant clinic."

"Here are those records, Doctor. Do you recognize them?"

"Yes, these are the clinic records."

"And those progress notes bearing your name were signed by you?"

"Yes, they were."

"I call your attention to the very last progress note, Doctor. Please read it for me."

"Continues to have diffuse left upper quadrant pain, anorexia, and weight loss. Joint pains continue and liver function tests getting worse. Will increase KZ67 and start on five milligrams of Prednisone daily. Previous diagnosis of hepatitis led to hepatic failure and liver transplant."

"Alright, now why did you start Prednisone and increase the KZ67?"

"She was showing signs of rejection, and that's the way we treat it."

"Really? How do you know she didn't have hepatitis?"

Swenz was rapidly becoming irritated with the inquisition. "I am the doctor, and I knew what her problems were! I don't see the need for me to have to explain myself to you, sir. I am the doctor!"

"While that may be true, I am entitled to ask the question."

"Please Doctor, answer it the best you can," pleaded Bert Rawley. Swenz sulked in his chair. The room had an eerie silence until he finally spoke. "The lab tests told me she was in rejection."

"Doctor, what is KZ67?"

"It is an anti-rejection drug we use to prevent rejection of a donor organ."

"Who is the manufacturer of this drug?" Swenz smiled as he leaned forward in anticipation of his answer. Now it was his turn. He would get even with them all, and he was just starting. "The drug is manufactured by Bently Drug Company."

"Is this an FDA-approved drug?"

"No, I don't believe it is."

"Is it an approved drug for clinical trials?"

"No, it isn't."

"Well sir, just how does such a drug become the mainstay of treatment in transplant patients?"

"The company made a deal with TWMC, Genome Corporation, and World Health HMO to conduct clinical trials on this research drug that had been found to work in other primates."

The court reporter raised her eyebrows in surprise and Nichols looked at Rawley in amazement. Rawley responded with a shrug of his shoulders and a slight turn of his neck.

"Off the record, please. May I speak with you a moment, Mr. Rawley?" He stood up and led the way out of the conference room into his private offic,e where he closed the door behind Rawley. "What are we getting into here, Bert?"

"This is the first I have heard this scenario. I'm as surprised as you."

"I never expected to get into anything like this but I am going to continue so that it's on the record. No doubt from what you told me last week about your client, the medical board will want to get their hands on this deposition."

"Do whatever you need to. My concern is the civil suit only."

Swenz was reliving his testimony and feeling very pleased with himself about the shrewd manner in which he'd implicated the conspirators.

"Back now on the record," announced Nichols.

"Doctor, before we broke, you were telling us about how KZ67 came about to be used at TWMC. How do you know all this to be a fact?"

"Well for one thing, I have been to the Research Lab in Malibu and I saw the manufacturing process at that time."

"What is the Research Lab?"

"It is the joint venture of Bently and Genome, as well as TWMC and World Health Care."

"Who was there at the time?"

"Michael Rome, CEO of Genome; Paul Cook, MD, chief

of Genome research; and Victor Matson, chief of Bently's research program."

"Anyone else?"

A large smile of satisfaction spontaneously appeared on his face.

"Yes. I was there with Doctor Sharon Dell."

"Who is she?"

"She is one of the lead transplant surgeons at TWMC."

"And she also witnessed that the drug was made at that facility?" Swenz was now euphoric and having difficulty holding back his eager responses until Nichols had finished with his question.

"She sure did, as a matter of fact, she was also a witness with me to the rest of the lab's secrets."

"Secrets? What do you mean, Doctor?"

"I mean that not only were they not FDA approved for the KZ67 clinical use, but they were also not approved for the genetic engineering or cloning of organs."

"I don't understand what you mean. Could you elaborate for us?"

"I'd be happy to, sir. You see, the four of them were in cahoots in everything developed by the lab. They had developed a remarkable genetic engineering process by which it became possible to clone any organ or body part from the patient's own blood cells. The genetic complement or DNA was used to grow the organs and ..."

"What? Are you telling me that the lab grew livers and kidneys and such?"

"Not only that, but also arms and legs that we transplanted

onto accident victim's bodies. They supplied the world market with cloned organs. They also developed the hepatitis D2 antigen against the virus that has ravaged the world. You see, they made fortunes through their discoveries but couldn't await FDA approval for the organs because the market forces throughout the world were demanding that they send in the clones!"

"I am going to leave this line of questioning for now. Doctor, did you examine Mrs. Firestone on that last visit?"

"No, I don't believe I did."

"And why not?"

"I didn't think it would be fruitful."

"I see. What if you had and discovered she had a massively enlarged spleen?"

"So what?"

"What training have you had in pediatrics, nephrology, cardiology, and gastroenterology, Doctor?"

"No specific training, but as a physician, I have been exposed to all of them."

"Are you trained and qualified to manage liver failure?" "I would ask for a consult."

"Are you sufficiently trained and qualified to evaluate a patient for the presence of liver failure?"

"That depends where they are in the stage of the disease."

"So you admit that there might be some stages of the illness that you wouldn't be able to detect yourself?"

"That's right. I would refer the patient ..." He stopped. He had been led into the trap, and the spring had been sprung. He had admitted that there were times when an expert in an area outside his specialty would be necessary to render proper care to a patient.

"Do you have any knowledge of the disease autoimmune hepatitis?

"Not much. It's one of those weird diseases."

"Yes, it is. As a matter of fact, it was the disease that caused the death of Sandra Firestone."

Swenz looked shocked. "That can't be!"

"I'm afraid it can, Doctor, and you missed the diagnosis. The autopsy revealed that she had recurrent chronic active hepatitis which, by the way, was the type of hepatitis that led to the need for her first liver transplant. Are you familiar with the treatment for this disease?"

"No."

"High doses of Prednisone, not five but fifty milligrams daily, along with with Immuran daily. Do you know what the chances of causing remission in her would have been had she been treated appropriately?"

"Twenty percent?"

"No Doctor, more like ninety percent, and she would be alive today if the diagnosis had been made timely, say six months ago when she started to have changes in the liver tests that you thought were due to rejection. Her arthritis pains were also quite typical of that diagnosis, my medical experts tell me. What do you think the cause of death was?"

"Liver failure?"

"No Doctor, the pathologist found she died of a splenic rupture. She had a subcapsular bleed of the spleen that was at least a month old. Do you think you might have found that if you had examined her?"

"I don't know."

"My medical experts tell me that any fall could have caused the bleed. As you know, when the spleen bleeds and its strong fibrous capsule remains intact, the bleeding remains confined to the organ and the patient has left upper quadrant pain. By the way, the reason she had a massive spleen was that her recurrent hepatitis led to portal hypertension, which precipitated the vomiting of blood on the day she died, as well as the secondary hypersplenism. You are familiar with that of course, aren't you?" he asked caustically.

Swenz sat in silence, stunned by the facts.

"Perhaps now you don't feel quite so qualified to manage the array of transplant patients? That will be all for now, Doctor, but I do reserve the right to recall you for a further deposition in the future."

– 38 –

SUSPICION
LOOMS HEAVY

Detective Tom Gray sat at his desk and shook his head. He'd been notified by Sharon and Michael that they needed to meet with him to give important information concerning an attempted murder. He listened to Sharon as she told her story of how she had been given the viral injection by Swenz and of the injections she'd then given to Gail and Ginny. Michael related the rest of the scenario and produced signed statements by Doctor Jack Kohl at the University Cancer Genetics Laboratory. They certified that all three cancers were derived from the oncogene found in the vial that Swenz had given to Sharon after he had injected her with some of its contents. He concluded with the facts surrounding Swenz's medical license suspension.

"Aren't you the doctor that filed a complaint with us about an attempt made on your life at the Olympics last year?"

Shocked at hearing the question, she gasped. "Why yes, I am."

"Is it possible that our good Doctor Swenz might have had something to do with it?"

Sharon turned pale, and she held her head with her hands, looking at the floor. "My God, do you think so?"

"Sounds like it might be possible. I need your signature on the complaint and I'll be paying him a visit very soon."

"Thank you, Detective. Call us if you need anything else." Michael and Sharon walked out of the San Bernardino Police Station hand-in-hand, feeling a load had been removed from their lives.

The next morning, Detective Gray and his partner paid a visit to the home of Barry Swenz. Gray rang the doorbell and they both waited patiently for the door to open. After a minute, it did.

"Doctor Swenz?" inquired Gray.

"Yes, I am Detective Gray and this is Detective Jenkins." Swenz became pale as the blood drained from his face. "How may I help you officers?"

"We need you to accompany us to the station so we can ask you some questions, sir."

"Fine with me. I'm ready."

They accompanied him to their car, where Swenz was placed in the back with Detective Jenkins. Strangely, Swenz didn't question why he was being brought in. He was too angry to think rationally. They drove to the station and went to a small room on the second floor, which had a small table and four chairs. The room resembled those Swenz had seen many times in cop movies. "So this is where you sweat the suspects."

"Have a seat, Doctor."

"What's this all about?"

"Doctor, you have the right to remain silent. Anything you say can and will be used against you in a court of law. You have the right to an attorney and, if you can't afford one, the State will provide one for you. Do you understand?" Gray was solemn.

"Of course I do. I have nothing to hide."

"Doctor, we are concerned about an incident that occurred at TWMC with Doctor Sharon Dell a few months ago."

Swenz began to sweat, and his tongue was feeling like cotton. "I don't know what you are talking about."

"Doctor Dell told us you gave her a hepatitis injection."

"I don't remember doing that." His hands were now clammy, and he felt his heart race. Swenz had already figured out a foolproof way to avoid answering questions about the hepatitis vaccine injection. It was simple, he calculated—he would deny ever having done it. What could they prove? If he said he didn't do it, it was his word against hers. He took certain solace in the fact she had already developed the cancer, but he had no knowledge of the newest developments that Sharon and the others were now rallying in their fight to kill the dreaded malignancy. He smiled at the policemen.

"Did you ever have in your possession a small vial of clear liquid that was labeled hepatitis D2 antigen?"

"I don't know what you are talking about," he responded smugly.

"Did anyone from the Research Laboratory in Malibu ever give you any small vial of fluid?"

"No, never." His mind drifted back to the event. He had discussed the snoopy Sharon Dell and her father with Michael Rome. Michael told him he would take care of Karl Dell and had indeed arranged for the public health nurse to administer the live hepatitis virus to cause the severe hepatitis and eventual liver failure. Rome had delivered the vial of live attenuated adenovirus with its deadly DNA oncogene load when they had met for dinner.

"Did you go to the Olympics last July, Doctor?" asked Detective Jenkins.

"No, I didn't."

"Do you have a good relationship with Doctor Dell?"

"I think so. We work together and often we share the same patients."

"Have you ever been angry at her?"

"No, not really."

"Do you recall confronting Doctor Dell in front of the sixth floor elevators one morning some months ago?"

"I don't recall."

"It had to do with a patient's care. Evidently, Doctor Dell instructed her resident to do something which was in contradiction to your orders."

Swenz sat at the desk with his right elbow on the table and his right hand on the right side of his face, trying to appear bored. He stroked his chin with his right hand as if in deep thought. "As I recall, we had a minor dispute about a patient care issue. That's all."

"Did you raise your voice at all in the dispute?"

"No, I didn't."

"What if we told you we had two witnesses who over-heard your dispute?"

"So what?"

"Well, would that change your testimony about raising your voice?" Barry thought a moment and thought they were bluffing about witnesses, because he hadn't noticed any at that time. "No, it wouldn't change my story at all."

"Doctor, we are going to release you, but you are not to leave town."

"What do you mean by that?"

"You are a suspect in the attempted murder of Sharon Dell."

"You can't be serious? What do you mean?"

"I can't divulge anything until we clear up a few matters first. We will be in touch with you. And by the way, since your medical license has been suspended temporarily, I assume we can reach you at home?"

Swenz stared at the detective with disdain and briskly walked out of the room.

– 39 –

ON THE MERITS OF
THE ACCUSATION

The day started off badly for Swenz in Judge Adam Kelly's
courtroom. The judge had admonished Barry that if he
heard one more outburst he would be evicted from the rest
of the hearing. Swenz sat down and fumed over the admoni-
tion. After a few minutes, his anger changed to pouting. The
State's witnesses provided brief, limited testimony, thus narrowing the scope for cross-examination. The State finished in
a record time of one hour and ten minutes.

The defense's case was over in twenty minutes. Sharon
testified to the personality changes she had witnessed in
Swenz and also delivered pleading testimony in support of
the transplant program. Further testimony was given by the
DOC and the medical board that TWMC had indeed closed
all the loopholes and corrected all the deficiencies that had
endangered patient care. They were satisfied TWMC had improved their quality of care.

"The court finds that Doctor Swenz's medical practice

is an extreme departure from the standard and there is sufficient evidence for the court to conclude he is suffering from a behavior disorder that requires medical and/or psychiatric treatment. Doctor Swenz's license to practice medicine in the state of California is suspended forthwith and he is ordered to seek full psychiatric evaluation and appropriate mental health treatment. The court further finds that the charges filed against TWMC are dropped on the basis of insufficient evidence presented by the State for a finding of neglect or willful misconduct."

The judge looked at Assistant A.G. Braun. "Will you prepare the minute order and have it on my desk this afternoon so I may sign it today?"

"Yes your Honor, I will."

Barotta peered at his client, Barry Swenz, who was staring into space. "Doctor, I'm sorry. You know, if you complete the psychiatric care, the medical board can be petitioned after three years to re-open your case. It is possible you could get your medical license back again at that time."

"What am I going to do in the meantime?"

"I really don't have an answer for you."

"I have to support myself." Barry was really thinking about the debt he owed his friends in Las Vegas. He knew he was at the end of their mercy. Thinking about the possibilities, he shuddered.

"Well, at least you're not going to jail."

"I guess that's a consolation." They walked out of the courtroom together. Sharon had left earlier with her father in order to avoid a confrontation with Swenz. Barry went directly home and started to pour himself a drink. He sat down and stared at the clear liquid nestling against the ice in the tumbler. He swirled the glass, gulped down its contents, set it on the table, and poured another. He had to figure it all out again. First, there was the loss of his medical license. Then there was the pending civil litigation against him for the wrongful death of Mrs. Firestone, where the suit was asking for a million dollars. Not to be underestimated was the recent investigation by the police stemming from charges brought by Sharon Dell against him for attempted murder. He was still feeling safe with regard to the latter because there was no proof, only her word against his. But now, what was his word worth? Not much, he thought—he didn't even have a work permit any more after today. He drifted into a deep sleep nurtured by the alcohol, coupled with depression gnawing at his soul. At first, the noise sounded like a tapping on a window, but it grew in intensity and became annoying as it rudely moved him into the here and now. He fought against being jarred from the blissful sleep where his problems had been expunged from his consciousness. "I'm coming," he shouted in the direction of the front door. Stumbling toward the abrasive knocking that had crescendoed, he arrived at the door. "Who is it?"

"Open up Doc, it's Randy from Vegas." The stark terror ran through his body like a knife. Barry quickly realized that the end had come and reluctantly opened the door. There stood Randy, all six feet, 250 pounds. He walked inside and sat down in the living room chair. "Well Doc, you got the money?"

"Randy, please, give me a break, I need more time to get it!"

"Sorry Doc, I got my orders from the big boss. He says if there's no dough, I got to convince you to get it."

"Randy, remember when you tried to kill Sharon Dell and you screwed it up miserably in Atlanta? I convinced your boss to leave you alone. You know I paid twenty thousand dollars to your boss for you to do that job, and he was sure I was going to demand a refund of sorts. He was going to put you away for the blunder, but I intervened and told him he could keep all the money. I saved you! You owe me, Randy. Just a few more days. I'll have the $30,000 the day after tomorrow, honest."

"Can't do it, Doc. I got to do what I got to do." His smile conveyed an evil intention that was more than apparent to Swenz. Barry's mouth and tongue were stuck together while his heart pounded. He thought of his body's own physiologic response to the fear and knew he had only one chance if he was to save himself.

He busted through the front door, slamming it shut on his assailant's hand as he attempted to keep the door from closing. Swenz knew he was in good shape because he jogged daily, but now he would need more than a jog if he was to escape. He ran as fast as he could down the street to the corner, then bolted through a backyard, crisscrossing a few streets until he entered the Walmart parking lot. He quickly darted inside the store. Impatiently, he looked outside the entrance for evidence that he had been followed. When ten minutes finally elapsed, he walked outside in his newly purchased sweatshirt and hat in a feeble attempt to disguise himself. Rapidly, he walked to the bus stop, then caught the bus to TWMC where he got off and walked inside. It was funny, he thought, how he felt so at home and safe at TWMC. His whole life had been so entrenched there for years, he knew no other home.

In the lobby, he went to the telephone and placed a call. "Hello, Mr. Jason Nichols please, this is Barry Swenz." The phone was silent. Nichols was amazed to receive a call from a party he was suing in a wrongful death action.

"Doctor Swenz, I am shocked you would call me. What do you want?"

"What I need to tell you has to be done in private. Can you meet me at TWMC? I'll be waiting in front for you. Just drive up to the front door and I'll be there." His voice was quivering now, making him sound very unstable. He knew it was because fear was causing adrenalin release.

"I don't know. I think I should talk to your lawyer first."

"Mr. Nichols, I am talking about a life and death situation! Please meet me. You have nothing to fear—I am the one who is in trouble."

"But … What about your attorney, Mr. Barotta? Why don't you call him?" "I don't have an attorney any longer. I fired him. He was being paid by TWMC to defend me before the medical board hearings."

"And Mr. Bert Rawlins, who represented you at the deposition?"

"Look, I don't have the money to pay for an attorney and I don't need one just to tell you a story you will definitely want to hear. I don't have much time, please."

"Perhaps you should call the police and talk with them?"

"I can't do that. There are other people after me, and if they found out I went to the police, my life wouldn't be worth a plug nickel. Look, if you refuse to meet me, you are the one who will lose out. I have some information I must give to you. An attack has just been made on my life. Please meet me."

Jason detected a sense of great fear in his voice. "Alright, I'll be there. His curiosity got to him and he felt compelled to find out what information Swenz had. It could help his client's case against TWMC, as well. After the knowledge that Swenz had imparted at the deposition, other pearls of wisdom might be gained. The more money in a judgment, the more there was for him. In any case, Jason figured that the good Doctor Swenz might end up being judgment-proof, which meant that there would be no source of payment. He had heard through the grapevine earlier that Swenz had lost his license and therefore couldn't practice medicine any longer. Without that license, Swenz's income would become nil. He had named TWMC in the action and therein lay his salvation. The medical center was the deep pocket, and now that he had evidence of the joint venture with the others, there loomed the potential of really big bucks. This was the kind of case every lawyer dreamed of. He needed as much information as he could collect for him to cash in for his client.

"Yes, I am on the way," Jason Nichols relented.

The car pulled up to the front of the hospital and Barry opened the door and slipped inside. He slouched down as Jason Nichols drove away. "There's a coffee shop at Central and Granger, let's go there."

They drove to the spot and both men walked in silence as they entered the brightly lit restaurant. Swenz removed his hat and sweatshirt and placed them on the seat next to him. He stared at Jason as the waitress approached. "What can I get for you?" she asked, looking at Barry.

"I'll have a cheeseburger, fries and coffee. Also bring me a green salad with Roquefort dressing, please."

"I'll have the same, but hold the salad."

When she left, Barry spoke.

"Mr. Nichols, what I am about to tell you may seem far-fetched and sound like science fiction, but I swear I am telling you the truth."

"I've come to hear your story, not to criticize it."

"Because I am a marked man, I truly believe I will be killed, and I have nothing to gain by lying to you. I want you to know the truth about this, so if something happens to me, you will be able to finger the culprits. They need to be reckoned with. Let me speak and then you decide."

"I've brought a tape recorder with me—do you mind if I record our conversation?" asked Nichols. Swenz thought a minute to himself and then responded. "As a matter of fact, I think it may be beneficial in the future. Go ahead and turn it on. You might want to say a few words at the onset to set the stage." The meal was set before them and they ate first. After they had finished eating, Jason placed the recorder on the table before them.

"I am Jason Nichols and I am here with Doctor Barry Swenz at six p.m. February 20 as he requested in a telephone call to my office at about five thirty today. He has agreed to allow this conversation to be taped." He motioned to Barry to continue.

"This is Barry Swenz speaking. I have given Mr. Jason Nichols my permission to tape this meeting. Some months ago, Doctor Karl Dell, Sharon Dell's father, became ill with the hepatitis D2 virus that destroyed his liver and caused the necessity for a liver transplant. The illness did not occur out of the blue. It was a preconceived, diabolical plan devised by Michael Rome."

"Who is he? I don't recognize his name."

"He's the CEO of Genome Corporation, the largest genetic research company in California, and probably the country. His corporation is in the joint venture partnership with Bently Drug Company, World Health Care, and TWMC."

"But how could anyone carry out such a scheme?"

"Simply. A nurse was sent by the Health Department to his office to immunize him against the hepatitis D2."

"Yes ..."

"She worked for Rome, and she injected him with live hepatitis D2 virus!"

"Why would he want to do that?"

"Because he wanted to cause the need for a liver transplant, and he wanted Sharon to owe him something."

"I don't understand."

"Look, Doctor Peter Halper, who works for Rome, discovered the process by which cells die. They developed a microchip that can be activated by the use of an electromagnetic pulse energy, which will cause his liver cells to produce a protein that signals for cell death. Their computer can track you anywhere in the world because the signal is bounced off a satellite."

"How can that affect him though?" he asked, looking in amazement at Swenz.

"Guess where the microchip is located?"

"Oh no! In his transplanted liver?"

"Right, and they can activate the chip to kill him any time they desire!"

Nichols's head turned from side to side in disbelief.

"Sharon Dell was told about this chip before the surgery, and that is what they are using to keep her from ever testifying against them on a myriad of issues she knows about."

Nichols's mouth fell open and he couldn't speak at first.

"I've got to hide out now. Can you let me have a few hundred dollars?"

Jason pulled out his wallet and handed Swenz four crisp one-hundred-dollar bills. This would have been cheap at twice the price, he thought. With this information, he might be able to get Sharon Dell to testify concerning juicy irregularities within TWMC that would convince a jury of their callousness and reckless disregard for the safety of their patients. No doubt, this would increase the award.

Swenz took the money and left the diner, while Jason sat in shock. Barry smiled to himself as he left and walked out into the street. "I'll nail TWMC. We'll see if they can escape from this now. Since they have plenty of money and are well insured by the same insurance company that I was with, they deserve to be screwed. They dropped me when I was a little late in payments; now it will cost them." Swenz was in his usual state of rationalization and fixing blame on others with a slight distortion of the facts so as to engender support for his irrational accusations in his own mind. He was now talking aloud to himself.

Ten minutes later, Jason paid the bill and drove back to his office. He placed a call to Sharon Dell, and Karl answered the phone.

"This is Jason Nichols, Doctor. I represent Mr. Firestone in the wrongful death suit against Doctor Swenz and TWMC."

"Yes, Mr. Nichols. How can I help you?"

"I have some very important information which I must talk to you about. Legally I can speak to you because you are not a party, nor are you involved in any way with my client's action. I want you to know that ethically, I am not supposed to speak with your daughter, but—if she were to be listening to our conversation, I wouldn't know it, would I?"

Karl wrinkled his brow and placed his hand over the mouthpiece of the phone. "Sharon, please pick up the extension and don't say anything. Mr. Nichols, the attorney, is on the phone. He would like you to hear what he is going to tell me, but he's not supposed to speak with you because of the suit against TWMC and Swenz." Sharon looked askance at her father and picked up the receiver.

"Mr. Nichols, go ahead. *I* am listening," said Karl.

"I have just had a meeting with Barry Swenz, where he told me of a sinister plot which was engineered by people you may know." Jason related the plan against Karl as he was told by Swenz.

"I can't believe what I've heard!" Sharon put her hand

over her mouth and looked at her father with widened eyes. She replaced the receiver on the cradle and sat down on the kitchen chair.

"After you have digested all of this, perhaps we can talk again. In the meantime, I strongly suggest you call the police and report this to them."

"Thank you for the information, sir. Good evening." He hung up the phone and walked into the kitchen.

"I don't know what to say, Dad. I had no choice but to operate on you or you would have died."

"Now, I am a walking time bomb ready to explode under the will of that sicko Rome."

They discussed everything Nichols had told him, and Sharon thought she would call Michael and see if he had any ideas.

When Michael arrived, Sharon explained everything to him in detail. He listened intently. "Before we go on Sharon, I have good news. The ultrasounds of your lymph nodes are all normal now, just like Ginny's and Gail's. I believe your cancer is completely gone. The virus with the p53 gene did the trick."

Karl hugged and kissed his daughter and held back tears. Sharon let out a huge sigh, releasing deeply pent-up emotions, and couldn't stop the laughter or the tears. They sat in silence, enjoying the moment. Michael broke the silence by asking Sharon, "What do you think about me calling Jack Kohl and getting his advice on this? Perhaps Jack has another such trick up his sleeve that we can use on Karl. Did you say

Doctor Peter Halper was responsible for the development of the microchip?"

"Yes."

▲ ▲ ▲

Jason Nichols had a lot to think about. Was he obliged to call the police about Swenz and report that he'd had an attempt made on his life? He pondered the question for a long while and came to the conclusion that he did have an obligation, as an officer of the court, to inform the authorities about the attempt. His motivation was also driven by the fact that he wanted a live witness to testify at the trial of his client because that was always more effective than a deposition, tape or affidavit. A jury would be inflamed by what Swenz had to say and, who knows, if Swenz came apart during testimony, there might even be more indictments of people in high places, whom the blame could be affixed upon. Nichols salivated at the prospect as he picked up the phone. He knew a few detectives on a first-name basis, and they might be interested in helping to save a life.

"Detective Crenna, please."

"Homicide, this is Detective Crenna speaking."

"Vinny, this is Jason Nichols. How are you?"

"Doin' fine, my main man, what gives?"

"I need a favor, Vinny." Jason told him about the attempt made on the life of Swenz.

"Did you say Doctor Barry Swenz, the orthopod at TWMC?"

"Yes, do you know him?"

"Know him? Why, one of the other detectives here just had him in for questioning on an attempted murder!"

"You mean he has reported this to you already?" Nichols said in disbelief.

"No, no, we brought him in for questioning because he is a suspect on another attempted murder case."

"You've got to be joking. What's it all about?"

"A lady Doctor at TWMC has filed a complaint. She alleges that he injected her with some kind of cancer-producing virus." Nichols sat in a stupor.

"Wait a minute. Let me check something with Detective Gray. Hey Tom, where are you with that Swenz case?"

Gray took his feet off the desk and wiped his lips. He swallowed the rest of the pie and turned his swivel chair to face Vinny. "We're waiting for some more lab reports, then we'll pick him up and charge him."

"You might never get the chance from what I hear."

"What?"

"My friend, an attorney, is on the line with a whale of a story. Pick up line three." Gray spun the chair around so that it almost did a 360 and caught the edge of his desk to stop the momentum. "Hello, Detective Gray here."

"Jason, Tom Gray is on the extension and he's in charge of the Swenz case. Tell him what you just told me." Crenna continued to listen to the conversation with interest.

Nichols reiterated the story told to him by Swenz.

"What kind of car was he driving?"

"He didn't have one. He ran from his house and I picked him up at TWMC. He didn't even have time to get his car.

"He must be going to a car rental agency then. We'll get on it right away. Thank you for the information, Mr. Nichols—you have been very helpful."

"Will you pick him up now?"

"You bet we will. He has now confessed to the attempted murder of Sharon Dell, and you have it on tape. We are about to charge him with a felony and we want him alive. We know that he is in deep trouble with the Las Vegas boys, and they don't fool around when they want to make a point."

"Okay—if I hear any more, I'll get back to you."

They hung up the call.

"Vinny, do me a favor and run a check on all the local car rental agencies and see what you can turn up."

"Sure thing, Tom," said Crenna. A few minutes later, he hung up and said, "Bingo. The Raleigh Hotel Avis Car Rental. He just drove away five minutes ago. The agent said he asked for a freeway map to take him to Newport Beach."

– 40 –

SAFE AT LAST

Barry Swenz had taken a cab to the Raleigh Hotel, where he found the Avis Rental Car Agency still open for business. He used his Mastercard to rent the car and drove away, headed west toward Newport Beach. He hadn't been there in more than five years. He looked at the map again and noted that he could hop on the 215 southbound and pick up the 91 that headed west toward Anaheim, but he would change onto the 55 south and then on to Newport Beach, where he would find a place to hide while he tried to sort things out. "It shouldn't take more than an hour and a half," he thought aloud. Careful not to attract any attention, he kept to the inside lanes and traveled no more than sixty miles per hour.

Detective Gray had issued an all points bulletin that notified all law enforcement agencies that Swenz was wanted for attempted murder and requested that the Highway Patrol set up roadblocks at the strategic intersections of the freeway route to Newport Beach. With the freeway map in front of him, he spoke with the highway patrol duty officer. "I believe he will head down the 91 to the 55. That seems like the most direct route. You may be able to pick him up at the ramp leading onto the 55 in about 45 minutes or so. Can you put up a block there and try to apprehend him for us?"

"We'll sure give it a try. And I'll call you later if we get him."

"Thank you. I'll be here waiting."

Swenz was driving along, listening to music, thinking about the tangled web he was in the midst of. The only thing that he felt good about was blowing the whistle on the joint venture conspiracy. He rapidly approached the intersection of the southbound 55 Freeway and was met by a stream of red lights in front of him. At long last, the bumper parade seemed to be at an end. There was one car in front of him that was stopped by a highway patrol officer. *I wonder what's going on here*, he thought as his car crawled to the officer and stopped. The officer was speaking into his microphone pinned to his shirt as he drew his nine millimeter and pointed it at Barry. He walked to the car. "Sir, please step out of the car."

Shocked at the confrontation, Swenz asked what he had done.

"Sir, please open the door and step outside," repeated the officer.

"I haven't done anything! What is all this about?" he asked in a raised, excited voice. He opened the door and stood facing the officer.

"Doctor, turn around and face the car and put your hands behind your back," came the order.

Stunned at the development, Swenz complied with the order and was immediately placed in handcuffs and taken into custody. Notice was given to Detective Tom Gray that Swenz was in custody and on the way back to San Bernardino. Swenz was charged with attempted murder of Sharon, Ginny, and Gail.

▲ ▲ ▲

Michael, Sharon and Karl were deep in thought. Michael finally spoke.

"We need to find out how the chip causes the cells to die. If we can get that information, we may have a chance at finding a way to prevent it from progressing to that point!" They all thought about it for a while, and then Sharon said, "Since Mr. Nichols was able to get this information in the first place, what about asking him to inquire through Swenz about the method. At least let's see what else he knows that might prove useful."

"Good idea, Sharon. I'll call him now," replied Michael.

"Mr. Nichols, this is Doctor Michael Herbert. I am a close friend and the treating physician of Doctor Sharon Dell. She asked me to see her father, Karl, and he has told me of the awful events you related to him leading to his liver transplant. I desperately need to find out more information on how the chip causes the cells to die. Evidently, Doctor Peter Halper was instrumental in this regard, and he would be the one to give me the answers I need to prevent a catastrophe from happening to Karl. Can you help?"

"I sure can try, but I don't know where to reach Swenz."

"Anything you can do will be greatly appreciated. Thank

you." Nichols hung up and sat at his desk with both hands holding up his face. He placed a call to the police and asked to speak with Detective Crenna.

"Hi Jason, back so soon. Have you got more news for us?" Quickly, Nichols repeated the request and concern for the information to his friend. "Can you try to find Swenz and get more information for Doctor Herbert?"

"You must live right, old man—Swenz was just brought in and is now being booked. I'll get on it right away."

He hung up the phone and turned his seat around to face his friend. "Hey Tommie, guess what?" He relayed the desperate request to Tom Gray, who went to the lockup unit and spoke with Swenz. He then returned to his desk and asked Crenna to accompany him on a visit.

"Where are we going?"

"We are going to pay a visit to a Doctor Peter Halper at his home. I have a number of questions to ask him that were faxed to me by Doctor Herbert. I don't understand them, but evidently it's critical information that the doctor must have in order to save a patient's life."

$-41-$

SOLUTIONS AT HAND

M rs. Halper graciously led Gray and Crenna into the living room and asked them to be seated while she retrieved her husband. In a few moments, Doctor Peter Halper appeared and approached his visitors with hand outstretched. Gray introduced Crenna and himself and sat down. "I won't waste your time, sir—we will be brief. We need to ask you some questions."

"I'll help you, if I can."

"You are employed by the Research Laboratories in Malibu, aren't you?" asked Gray opening his small notebook to a fresh page.

"Why, yes, I am. I have been employed there for almost six months now," came the response in a matter-of-fact fashion.

"Doctor, I am not going to beat around the bush. We have certain evidence that links you with a conspiracy plot to injure Doctor Karl Dell."

Halper blanched at hearing Gray's statement. "I don't know what you mean!"

"We have your fingerprints on a vial from your lab labeled *hepatitis D2 Vaccine*. In reality, the vial contained a potentially deadly virus that caused three women to develop cancer. Now, you can come clean and answer our questions truthfully, and we won't press charges of conspiring to murder Sharon Dell and two other women, or you can refuse to answer, and we'll go to the station and book you for the crime." Halper's head dropped, and he felt as if all the strength had ebbed from his body. He sat motionless for a few minutes, conscious of his unexpected visitors' eyes intensely trained upon him.

"What will I be charged with?" asked Halper softly.

"That will be up to the DA, but I'd guess that you would be charged with being an accessory, which is a much lesser felony. I assure you, we will make certain the DA is informed that you have cooperated with us in this matter. His word will go a long way with the judge and will be very important in the sentencing aspect of the trial. I can assure you there will be a trial, and, very soon. Doctor Swenz is already in custody and has told us a great deal about the Research Laboratory and the conspiracy perpetrated against Doctors Sharon and Karl Dell."

"Okay, I was involved ..."

"Hold it there, Doctor, I am going to tape your statement." He withdrew a small tape recorder from his pocket and placed it next to Halper. "This is Detective Tom Gray at the home of Doctor Peter Halper. Detective Victor Crenna is also present, and Doctor Halper has agreed to allow us to tape his statement. He has been Mirandized and wishes to proceed at this time without the benefit of an attorney present. Isn't that true, Doctor?" "Yes, I have agreed to give this statement myself without counsel present and I agree to the taping. Shortly after I became employed by the Research Labs, I was approached by Michael Rome, the CEO of Genome Corporation. He asked me about the research I had just published on cell death. One thing led to another, and before long, he asked me if a mechanism could be developed to trigger the process by using a microchip. He knew that I had been a pioneer in that exact research and had developed the technique by which a GPS could be used for that purpose. I told him I had already devised and tested such a device in animals. He offered me a bonus of $150,000, tax free, if I would agree to allow the microchip to be used in a human. He then told me about Karl Dell and why he wanted to use it. He needed to ensure the silence of Sharon Dell concerning the cloning of organs."

"Whoa, what's that about organ cloning?"

"The lab had developed the process of cloning organs and growing them like vegetables in a garden for prospective transplant patients." Gray looked at Crenna and squinted his eyes at hearing this description. Crenna returned the incredulous look with a shrug of his shoulders.

"Why did Rome want to be certain Sharon Dell remained silent?"

"Because the genetic process was not FDA approved. They were selling the cloned organs to the rest of the world, and evidently, there were no significant problems with them that I knew about. Doctor Dell was made aware of this fact and she agreed to continue the surgery transplantation. However,

Rome was still kind of paranoid about her and needed assurance that she would not blow the whistle on them, because they were making a fortune on it. By having the microchip in place, we could activate it with our computer, and that threat was used to keep her silent. We met with her at Spago right before her father's liver transplant and disclosed this to her. She became very angry, but nevertheless, she had no choice but to transplant the liver with the chip into her father. A refusal to do so would have sealed Karl's fate." Detective Gray pulled a paper from his pocket and read it.

"Can you write down all the facts that reveal how you activate the cellular death?"

"Yes," replied Doctor Halper.

"I need you to show all the molecular and cellular chemistry," said Gray reading from the paper.

"Yes, I'll do that now. May I use your notebook?" Gray handed it to Halper, who immediately began to write out the mechanisms. When he finished, he handed it back to Detective Gray.

"Thank you, Doctor. You have been very helpful, and let's hope you have also been instrumental in saving Karl Dell's life. That will look good for you with the judge. We will be in touch with you. Do not tell anyone we have been here."

"I understand." He got out of his chair and led them to the door.

Upon returning to the station, Gray phoned Michael to get his home fax number. Gray made a copy of his notebook pages containing the writings of Doctor Halper and faxed them to Michael, who was elated when he read what Halper had written.

The meeting was at Doctor Jack Kohl's office at University Hospital Genetics and Cancer Research Laboratory. Michael, Karl and Sharon were seated at a table in a small conference room where they were all sipping steaming coffee from a variety of mugs. It was painfully obvious that the major drug companies had found their way into Jack's secret den.

"It amazes me to see the amount of money these companies spend on gimmicks," said Michael, pointing to his own large mug endorsed with the name of a newly released antibiotic. "I'll get right to the point, Jack. First, Sharon, Gail and Ginny are all completely healed. I cannot find any sign of residual cancer. All tests are negative."

"That's wonderful news, Sharon," he said, looking at her.

She smiled back and interjected, "I owe you my life. I can't thank you enough for what you have done for the three of us." She smiled at him, and Jack was flattered by the comment.

"We have seen the same results in other similar cases where we unleashed the effects of a suppressor gene." "You did so well, Jack, that we have come back with another problem we all hope you can help us with."

"I'm flattered. Please go on." Michael repeated the entire story about Karl Dell's hepatitis and the transplanted liver that contained the microchip which controlled the "Sword of Damocles." He then gave him the statement written by Doctor Halper. Jack smiled as he read the notes.

"This is amazing," he said, "Halper's research on cell

death is well supported by the literature but I hadn't realized that he had developed a method by which he could trigger the process by an electromagnetic force. To control it by computer accessing the GPS via satellite is truly a stroke of genius.

"You know that one of the research projects we have been working on is also apoptosis. We know that the capacity for a cell to kill itself is essential to health. Normal cells are programmed with a definitive life span and are killed to make room for new cells. The abnormal function of apoptosis, which may end up causing excessive or even not enough cell death, may be the cause of diseases like Alzheimer's, rheumatoid arthritis, and cancer. The Greek word apoptosis means a dropping off and is pronounced *app-oh-toe-sis*, the second p remains silent. Various external and internal stimuli may trigger cell death, which is tempered by the Bcl-2 protein and its family of molecules. They are the Bax proteins, which promote apoptosis or prevent it, depending upon their concentrations within the cell.

"We have recently been involved with viral relations. It seems that when the apoptosis regulations become disturbed, viruses can be affected. After a virus enters a cell, it tries to stop the cell from making any other protein except those needed to help the virus reproduce. Many of the host cells will die, and so will the virus. Over time it appears that the Epstein-Barr virus that causes infectious mononucleosis has achieved a way to make certain proteins. As a matter of fact, the EB virus makes a protein similar to Bcl-2 which, when present in excess of Bax, inhibits the initiation of apoptosis.

It can also produce certain substances that cause the host cell to increase its own production of Bcl-2. The p53 apoptosis inducer can be inactivated by some viruses also. It seems to me that the most direct route to prevent the microswitch from initiating apoptosis might be to use the Epstein-Barr virus that has had its virulence attenuated. We can inject it into Karl's liver directly."

Karl winced at hearing this treatment offered by the expert and asked, "How would we do this?"

"We have done this in monkeys and in other mammals, but never in humans. It seems the virus production of Bcl-2 is stimulated maximally when the virus duplicates inside reticuloendothelial cells. If we inject the virus load by way of a biopsy needle, the virus will be deposited in close enough proximity to access the hepatic reticuloendothelial cells. They will produce the protein and, as long as they do, apoptosis can never begin."

"But how long will the virus continue to produce this protein? I sure don't want to have repeated liver injections as long as I live," said Karl, appearing extremely concerned at the prospect.

"That won't be necessary, because once the EB virus takes up residence, it's there for life, and the production of Bcl-2 will never stop, thereby maintaining a permanent shield of protection against the microchip action."

– 42 –

THE ROUNDUP

D etective Tom Gray presented his case to the DA, and requested that the DA obtain a subpoena from the judge
for all records of the Research Laboratories as well as all records of the joint venture. In that vein, a flurry of subpoenas
were issued to TWMC, Genome Corporation, Bently Drug
Company, and World Health Care HMO. Many lawyers suddenly found themselves engaged by wealthy clients who were
accused of grievous criminal acts.

At the arraignment hearing, TWMC was accused of
being in violation of the State Health and Welfare Code,
which mandated that all drugs and medications be approved
by the FDA. There were also the charges of conspiracy to
commit murder and the attempted murder of Doctors Karl
and Sharon Dell. Michael Rome and Genome Corporation
were accused of the same, as well as other violations of the
California Health & Welfare Code. David Malkin and Bently
Drug Company were also charged with the same violations.
World Health Care was charged with numerous violations of
the H&W Code along with violations of the Knox Keene

Law, which regulates the licensure of HMOs in the state of California. Doctor Peter Halper was charged as an accomplice in the attempted murder charges, and Doctor Barry Swenz was charged with the attempted murder of Sharon and Karl, but no charges were levied against him for H&W Code violations, since that had been previously adjudicated by Judge Adam Kelly.

The trial was to be held in the San Bernardino County Superior Court and, during the two months awaiting the trial, a number of extremely interesting things occurred. When Rome got wind of the impending indictments that the grand jury had handed down, he called Sharon Dell in order to explain his position to her.

"Dr. Dell, I suppose this call is superfluous, but I will feel better after we have a little talk."

"We are not talking about anything, Mr. Rome."

"Need I remind you that I hold the key to your father's life," he asked sarcastically.

"And need I remind you that you are attempting to blackmail me! And furthermore, I have it on good authority directly from the office of the Attorney General of California, that you, sir, will be brought to justice for the insane attempt to kill me with cancer!"

Rome bit his lip with anger. "That is a lie! I knew nothing about Swenz's action." Secretly, he hoped to God that the State would never be able to prove their case. It was his word against Swenz's. *They will never take the word of a doctor whose license has been revoked against mine*, he thought. "If you testify against me, I promise you that your father's liver will die and soon."

"We shall see about that!" Sharon slammed the receiver down so hard that it bounced off and fell to the floor. She began thinking about her father's procedure, where the virus was introduced into his liver. Six weeks had passed since Karl had undergone the direct injection of the EB virus into his organ. Michael had performed the procedure at 8 a.m, and Karl had gone home at 4 p.m. the same day without any complications. Liver biopsy procedures had been around for thirty years or more and had a wide margin of safety. Karl felt at ease since this was his second one. It was an amazing accomplishment though, to be able to use the procedure to inject virus into the liver rather than to extract a small piece of liver tissue for examination. The long Menghini needle had to be inserted directly into the liver about three inches, using local anesthesia only. When the needle was imbedded in the liver, the syringe was pulled back quickly to create a suction effect, and then withdrawn completely. A core of liver tissue would then be found in the lumen of the needle and easily expressed by injecting saline into the needle, allowing the plug of tissue to fall into a waiting container of formaldehyde.

Karl had refused to take any intravenous Versed, which would have put him out for the few minutes required to perform the procedure. The interesting concept about pain from the procedure was that the only pain fibers other than those blocked by the Lidocaine local anesthetic were those that were in Glisson's Capsule, which covered the liver. The tough capsule was able to transmit pain but the liver itself was devoid of nerves to transmit pain. After the local was applied, Michael attached a syringe containing Lidocaine to the needle and slowly advanced it, injecting the anesthetic along the path. When he felt the resistance of the capsule, he stopped and filled a syringe once more with five milliliters of Lidocaine and swapped it for the empty syringe that was connected to the Menghini needle. He then injected the Lidocaine, thus anesthetizing the entire area.

"Karl, I am going to ask you to hold your breath in a moment. When I do, I will be advancing the needle into the liver and it will take me ten seconds to inject the virus, so don't move or we may cause a laceration to the liver. I am going to go through a dry run with you now."

"Fine, go ahead." Michael removed the now-empty syringe that had contained the Lidocaine and substituted the one containing one milliliter of virus suspended in saline. "Take a big breath in and blow it all out. Now hold your breath!"

He counted ten seconds and added three seconds for good measure.

"Breathe now, Karl.

"That was a piece of cake," said Karl. "I assume the breath is held at end exhalation so the liver is at the highest position with the diaphragm maximally elevated?"

"That's right, and now let's do the real thing. Remember not to move," Michael admonished. He advanced the long slender needle until he felt the resistance of the capsule. He noted that Karl showed no evidence of pain on his face. "Now hold your breath!"

He rapidly advanced the needle while pulling back on the barrel of the syringe, and just as quickly expressed the saline with the virus back into the hole in the liver he had just made with the needle. He was done in seven seconds. "You can breathe now. I am going to have you lie on your right side against these sand bags, Karl." With the procedure completed, he wrote the standard post-liver biopsy orders and told the nurse he would return in six hours to discharge his patient. Michael had learned from Jack Kohl that the virus should have easily accomplished its intended job by six weeks. The only problem with the presumption was that there was no way to verify it.

If the protein Bcl-2 was produced in excess of the BAX protein, the liver cells would live and the process of apoptosis would be prevented by the computer-generated electromagnetic signal directed at the fiendishly placed microchip. Since it had been proven to be effective in other mammals, Karl felt good about it, as did Sharon and Michael.

– 43 –

EVEN TRIALS
COME IN THREES

*T*his is really something, thought Swenz as he sat in his cell at the County Jail awaiting the criminal trial. He had just received a note from his attorney, Bert Rawlins, notifying him that he would be taken to court the next morning for the start of the civil trial for the wrongful death charges made against him by Mr. Firestone. *I have been through a trial for my medical license and lost that round, and while I am awaiting the criminal trial, I have to go to court on this crap.*

Presiding over the trial in San Bernardino Superior Court was Judge Harold Thompson. The opening statements were brief, and the plaintiff's attorney, Jason Nichols, made it clear that he was going after the deep pockets. He named TWMC, Bently, and Genome as the culprits who had knowingly conspired to allow a non-FDA-approved drug to be used on Mrs. Firestone. Hearing the attack on his former allies, Swenz was delighted, because it substantiated his position. He was going to blow them all out of the water, but to do it would take a bit of clever maneuvering. He couldn't show the jury he was eager or they might suspect his motive was revenge and not valid.

The plaintiff's case moved forward with ease for the first hour, and then he was on stage.

"Dr. Swenz, please take the stand." He rose and slowly walked to the witness stand and was sworn in.

Jason Nichols asked the usual preliminary questions to establish that Swenz had been an employee of TWMC and asked for a description of his duties.

"So, you personally attended the postoperative transplant patients for almost four years?"

"Yes."

"What training have you had in this area?"

"I am trained as an orthopedist and I received special training in the use of the anti-rejection drug KZ67 made by Bently Drug Company. I have had no other formal training."

"Have you been trained in pediatrics?"

"No."

"What about internal medicine or gastroenterology?"

"No."

"Have you received any training in any other area of medicine or surgery?"

"No."

"Is it proper for someone without formal training in a specialty to care for patients in an area where others more competent in that field are available?"

"No, it isn't." Nichols was stunned at the answer after the runaround he'd gotten from Swenz at his deposition.

But upon further recollection, he remembered the ease with which Swenz had also told him about the conspiracy against Karl and Sharon.

"Doctor, I am going to read your deposition aloud now." "You can save yourself a lot of time, Mr. Nichols. Mrs. Firestone died as a result of my failing to diagnose her recurrent chronic active hepatitis in a timely manner. I am truly sorry for my ignorance."

Bert Rawlins stood and proclaimed his objection. "Since Dr. Swenz wasn't an expert in liver disease and had never held himself out to be an expert in that area, his testimony should be struck for lack of foundation."

"Sustained."

Swenz was happy. At least he had given the jury an admission of guilt to help them arrive at a verdict. He knew if he baited Nichols, he would attempt to show that he was an agent of a larger company and therefore they were just as responsible for the death of Mrs. Firestone as he was. He was well versed with the legal definition of agency in California law, because many years ago, he had been sued for malpractice. He'd been working for another doctor and had misdiagnosed a problem in a patient. Since he was an employee and was required to do everything according to his employer's wishes, the court had found that he was indeed an agent of his employer, so the employer was also found liable on the legal theory of agency.

"Dr. Swenz," began Nichols, "can you change your own schedules?"

"Not usually. Only if an emergency occurs."

"Are you required to follow a set pattern of work?"

"Yes."

"Could you have refused to see the post-transplant patients and refused to treat them with the KZ67?"

"No."

"And why was that?"

"Because there was no one else to do it. If I had refused, they would have fired me." He knew that was what Nichols really wanted to hear.

"So to recap, all surgery and clinic patients were scheduled by others and you had no authority to alter those schedules?"

"Correct."

"How did you alter the dosage of the KZ67 drug?"

"I don't understand the question."

"Did you decide on the revised doses based upon your interpretation of the lab tests and your own choice of the dosage?"

"Oh no! Bently gave me their protocol to follow, and I did just that."

"Do you now hold a valid medical license to practice in the state of California?"

"Objection, Your Honor. This has nothing to do with the issues at hand," said Bert Rawlins.

"On the contrary," responded Nichols. "May we have a sidebar, Your Honor?"

"Certainly." The judge motioned to the court recorder to join them. "What is going on here?" he asked.

"I have the right to show that the doctor has lost his license to practice," explained Nichols.

"That is not the subject of this trial. It has nothing to do with what he is alleged to have done."

"In view of the doctor's recent testimony, I don't believe that *alleged* is the proper word now," quipped the DA.

"That testimony was stricken," replied the judge.

"By showing that the medical board has revoked his license for gross incompetence, I am getting validation of his poor performance on Mrs. Firestone." "I am not going to allow you to proceed along this line of questioning, Mr. Nichols, because of the relevance issue as I see it. I will, however, allow you to call the medical board as a witness, but their testimony is restricted to any reviews on the care of Mrs. Firestone they have personal knowledge of."

"I have spoken with Doctor Gannon of the medical board and he has told me that Dr. Swenz's continued use of a non-FDA approved drug and his willingness to practice in areas he had no training in have been found by the board to represent an extreme departure from the standard of practice. They did not specifically review any of Mrs. Firestone's chart at that time."

"Then, that settles it. You can't bring him in as a witness," said Rawlins.

"They did get testimony at the ISO hearing from Doctor Dell that Swenz tried to kill her with an injection of a virus that caused her to develop cancer."

"That should not be allowed into evidence, Your Honor," pleaded Rawlins. "It bears no relevance again."

"I am going to sustain Mr. Rawlins's objection. Mr. Nichols, I will allow you to present any evidence that is specific to your client, but nothing about any of this peripheral stuff."

They returned to their positions, and Nichols looked at Dr. Swenz.

"Doctor, do you consider yourself a good physician?"

"Yes."

"Are you planning to return to TWMC to work?"

"No."

"And why not?"

"Because I don't have a license to practice anymore."

"Objection, Your Honor. I move to strike the defendant's testimony as non-responsive!"

"Sustained. Ladies and gentlemen of the jury, you are hereby instructed to disregard the last statement by the witness."

"That's all, Doctor. You're excused." He now had all he needed, even the fact that Swenz's license had been revoked.

Dave Malkin, CEO of Bently, testified that Swenz was never told what to do and how to do it. When he was shown the dosing schedule on his own stationery signed by the medical director of research, Doctor Victor Matson, he changed his story to the satisfaction of attorney Nichols. James Foxworthy admitted that Swenz was an employee of TWMC and their agent as well. Michael Rome's testimony revealed that there was a joint venture agreement that had been formed for the purpose of pooling resources to help in the development of the hepatitis D2 vaccine, the clinical trials of KZ67, and the genetic cloning of various organs and other body parts for application throughout the world.

Testimony from World Health Care HMO corroborated the previous facts set forth by the witnesses. Financial information revealed the hundreds of millions that were made by the consortium as well.

After a brilliant summation and closing statement, the jury was discharged to deliberate. It took them only two days to reach a verdict of guilty and to award the sum of two million dollars against each of the members of the joint venture and Doctor Swenz. They had also found, as requested by Nichols, that the verdict was joint and several, which meant that one or all of the defendants were liable for payment. Since Swenz had nothing, the judgment of ten million dollars fell upon the other four defendants to pay. Nichols was delighted because he now had not just one viable source to collect the judgment from, but four sources who were all very wealthy. This was California, and the state was well known for large plaintiff verdicts by liberal juries. Because of Swenz's inflammatory testimony on the tape given to them by Nichols, the DA's office filed charges against all of the joint venture partners for numerous criminal violations of the law as well as the attempted murder of both Sharon and Karl Dell.

~ **44** ~

THE FINALE

S wenz spent the next month in a happy mood behind bars, knowing that his former partners had been
nailed through his testimony. In jail, he had been visited by
Detectives Gray and Crenna to question him further about
the statements he had allowed Nichols to tape record. On
their last visit, they had told him about the criminal charges
that the DA had filed against his former partners.

The day had finally arrived for the criminal trial, and unknown to any of the defendants, a representative from the
federal attorney's office was present in the courtroom to evaluate the merits of the case for federal prosecution. The feds
had been notified by the California Attorney General's office
of potential federal HCFA violations by all the defendants.
Rather than waiting for the trial to conclude and waiting again
for a copy of the lengthy transcript, their interest was sparked
enough to assign one of their attorneys to observe the trial.

"All rise, the Honorable Jack Maloney presiding," barked
the bailiff. The shuffling of chairs was very apparent as the
attorneys scrambled to their feet. The judge peered over his

glasses at the packed courtroom and nodded at the bailiff, who walked to the door to the left of the bench and returned with Doctor Swenz dressed in a sport coat and tie. "The people versus Doctor Barry Swenz, TWMC, Genome Corporation, Bently Drug Company, and World Health Care HMO," said the clerk.

Opening statements were brief on both sides. It was made apparent that the DA's position was that Swenz was acting as an agent for the rest of the conspirator defendants. They were equally as guilty for the attempt to kill Sharon and her father. Other charges were that TWMC had violated the state's Title 22 law, which mandated certain safeguards and precautions be in place. Allowing Swenz to practice in areas he was not deemed to be proficient in and thereby endanger the lives of others, would not be difficult to prove. Michael Rome and his corporation were charged with attempted murder along with David Malkin and Bently. Conspiracy charges were also filed against Genome and Bently.

Swenz was feeling no anxiety about the trial. He still felt that no one could find him guilty of the crime he was charged with against Sharon. There were no witnesses, and his mind was filled with a self-assurance which alone was quite pathological.

"The people call Doctor Barry Swenz to the stand," said assistant district attorney Fred Acosta.

"Raise your right hand. Do you swear to tell the truth, the whole truth and nothing but the truth, so help you God?" asked the court clerk.

"I do."

Acosta slowly approached the witness stand and stared at Swenz. The court was silent for an unnerving minute.

"State your name and spell it for the court." Swenz responded to the command.

"Doctor, please give us a summary of your education and professional activities."

Swenz looked at his attorney, Lionel Grant, and rolled his eyes. *This is so dumb*, he thought. "I have repeated this litany in every trial thus far." Lionel nodded to his client in a silent mandate to conform with the request. Begrudgingly, Swenz methodically related his educational history and professional activities to the court.

"Doctor, did you immunize Doctor Sharon Dell against hepatitis D2 in the last nine months?"

"No." "Have you ever given her an injection of any type?" "No."

"What is your relation with Genome and Bently?"

"I have done work for them at TWMC. I was responsible for following the organ transplant patients and adjusting their anti-rejection drugs until they developed a revised drug that only had to be administered for a short period of time."

"Were you on their payroll as an employee?"

"No, I received payments as an independent contractor from their Research Laboratory."

"What evidence do you have to support that contention?"

"My bank deposits. Mr. Grant has my accounts." He pointed a finger at his attorney, who sat motionless at the defendant's table.

"May I approach the witness, Your Honor?"

"You may," responded Judge Maloney without looking up from his bench.

"Are these the checks that were issued to you and deposited?" he asked as he handed a pile of checks to Swenz. Barry looked through the pile and was amazed as he counted the total amount of money he'd been given over four years.

"Yes, these are the payments I received for my work."

"Tell us how much they total, please." There was a slight but obvious hesitation by Swenz.

"Eight hundred and seventy thousand dollars." A murmur could be heard coming from the court spectators.

"And over what period of time were those checks written?"

"Four years."

"Were you to receive any other money from them?"

"Yes. I was promised by Mr. Rome and Mr. Malkin that when the profits from the hepatitis D2 vaccine, the KZ67, and the FDA approval for the cloned organs came through, I would receive about twenty million dollars as my share."

"Did you also receive a salary from TWMC?" asked Acosta.

"Yes, I was paid two hundred thousand dollars per year."

"So then Doctor, if my math is correct, you received about $400,000 per year. Is that correct?"

"Objection. Relevance, Your Honor," stated Grant.

Acosta was quick to respond. "My line of questioning all has to do with motive."

"May we have a sidebar, please?" asked Grant. The judge signaled the court recorder to the bench.

"I intend to show that Doctor Swenz was motivated by greed flamed by a gambling addiction. The evidence will show he was easily bought by others who were all too eager to take advantage of the pressures he was under from his Las Vegas friends with regard to his gambling debts."

"I will allow the question to establish Doctor Swenz's state of mind during the last four years," ruled Judge Mahoney.

The trial continued.

"Doctor, how many dependents do you have?"

"Only me."

"What are your monthly expenses? As close as you can estimate."

"Seven to eight thousand dollars a month."

"Do you own any real estate other than your home?"

"No." "Do you have any savings?"

"No."

"Do you own any stocks or bonds?"

"No."

"Other than your car and home, do you own any other valuable items?"

"No."

"Well then, Doctor, where did all your money go? If we assume your taxes were about seventy-five thousand dollars per year and you spent eighty-five thousand dollars annually, that leaves almost a quarter million dollars unaccounted for."

"I gambled it all in Las Vegas." The courtroom murmur was now loud.

"Order in the court!" demanded the judge.

"So your salary at TWMC was used for your living

expenses exclusively, while the money you received from the Research Laboratory was used to finance your gambling habit. Isn't that true?"

"I guess that it is."

"Was there ever a time in the last four years that you were not in debt to Las Vegas gambling?"

"On occasion, I would be debtless for a month or so, but it was a rare occurrence."

"That will be all for now, Doctor."

"You may step down, Doctor, but remember that you are still under oath," cautioned the judge.

"The people call Doctor Sharon Dell to the stand."

Sharon walked to the witness stand, and when she had seated herself, raised her right hand. The defense stipulated to the prosecution receiving Sharon's curriculum vitae into evidence. The five-page document contained her entire educational and professional background, and her attestation to its veracity was accepted by the court.

"Doctor Dell, please tell us what your position is at TWMC."

For the next five minutes Sharon summarized her position and duties for the jury.

"What is your relationship with Doctor Swenz?"

"He is in charge of the Department of Orthopedics at TWMC. We had a professional relationship."

"What do you mean by had?"

"About eight months ago, he verbally assaulted me about the management of a patient. It was my position that the patient's orthopedic problem could have easily waited until the more pressing and potentially devastating problems were under control. It would have put the patient at too high a risk to undergo orthopedic surgery first. Doctor Swenz attacked me because I directed my resident, Doctor Evans, to cancel the surgery. He screamed and ranted at me in the hallway of the hospital."

"Was that the first time you noticed atypical behavior on his part?"

"I believe so."

"Tell us how you happened to visit the Research Laboratory in Malibu, California?"

"Doctor Swenz told me that he had been asked by Bently Drug Company to treat transplant patients with the anti-rejection drug KZ67. This drug was not FDA-approved. He told me that the researchers, who were world renowned, wanted to show me what research they had accomplished in that area so I agreed to go with him to visit the laboratory."

Sharon continued to relate the case of Linda Korn, which had started her thinking about everything. When she finished her testimony about that issue, she was then asked about the circumstances surrounding the almost fatal immunization she received at the hands of Swenz. She described every detail to the jury. "You looked at the label on the vial that Doctor Swenz brought to your office?"

"Yes, I did. It said 'hepatitis D2 Vaccine."

"Describe what happened then."

"Swenz took a syringe from his pocket and attempted to put the needle into the rubber vial cap to withdraw the fluid, but he inadvertently jabbed himself with the needle.

He discarded the needle and tried again with a new one. This time he withdrew the fluid and I allowed him to inject it into my right shoulder muscle, right here." She pointed to her right deltoid area.

"Alright, what happened after Doctor Swenz injected you with the vaccine?"

"I then asked him to leave the rest with me so I could immunize my clinical personnel. We were seeing many infected hepatitis D2 patients, and I wanted to give my people protection against contracting the deadly virus. He told me that we would not be receiving the vaccine for use in the hospital for a week or two. I immunized two women with the contents of the vial and put the rest in my top right desk drawer, which I've always kept locked. I am the only one with a key."

"What are the names of the two women?"

"Ginny Ross and Gail Poland."

"Please tell us what happened to Ginny, Gail, and yourself over the next eight weeks after you received the injection."

Sharon told about her mass in the axilla and those of Gail and Ginny. She then told of Doctor Michael Herbert's examination of all of them and the biopsy results.

"Would you relate the circumstances surrounding your father Karl Dell's illness?"

Sharon complied in meticulous detail and concluded with the details of the meeting at Spago, as well as Michael Rome's last threatening telephone call.

Acosta called attorney Nichols, who testified to his conversation with Swenz where he implicated the other conspirators and produced the tape for the jury to hear firsthand.

After the lunch break, Doctor Michael Herbert testified that he'd diagnosed cancer in all three of the women and his curiosity was piqued at the unusual presentation of the cancers and how the three women worked together. He related his discussions with his colleague and friend Doctor Jack Kohl, senior researcher at the University Cancer and Genetics Laboratory.

Throughout all the testimony Swenz laughed to himself. Where was the evidence against him? Who could possibly prove he had injected the cancer virus into Sharon? There were no witnesses. He took solace in that fact as he watched the proceedings.

"The people call Doctor Jack Kohl to the stand." He was sworn in and took his seat.

"Doctor, please summarize your educational training for us."

"Your Honor, the defense will stipulate to the Doctor's C.V. being introduced into evidence in order to save the court's time. I have read it and I agree he may be called as an expert witness."

The lengthy C.V. was carried to the court clerk, who announced that it was being identified as People's number 34.

"May I look at that please?" asked the judge. The clerk handed it to him upon hearing the request and returned to her desk.

"Please tell us where you are employed and what you do there."

"I have been employed by Southern California University School of Medicine for the last fifteen years in the Department of Cancer Genetics, where I am in charge of research."

"Have you published scientific papers, doctor?"

"I have published more than a hundred papers in the field."

"In what journals have you done so?" "Scientific American, Publications of the National Institute of Health, Current Opinions in Oncology, Cancer, Epidemiology of Cancer, American Journal of Public Health, Cancer Research, Cancer Epidemiology, Biomarkers and Prevention, and CA Cancer Journal for Physicians. I have written a textbook entitled *The Oncogene* as well as co-authoring many other articles and chapters of medical textbooks."

"Please tell us about your initial meeting with Doctor Herbert and Doctor Dell."

"They came to my office at the university and Doctor Herbert related his findings in Sharon Dell, Ginny Ross, and Gail Poland. He was trying to find a common denominator in the three cancers. They all began in the lymph nodes of the armpit, and all the women had negative studies for the presence of cancer in the breast, yet their lymph node biopsies all revealed breast cancer. This combination of a breast cancer spread to the nodes without any source of the primary cancer detected within the breast raised his suspicion that there might be something else afoot here, and I agreed with him. You see, he had previously sent me a cell culture of each woman's biopsied tumor that I had analyzed for its DNA component. I had just completed the analysis a few days prior, and when he showed up in the office, I assumed he was going to tell me that the hospital lab had erred in their identifying each specimen. The DNA verified my belief that they were all from the same source. He told me that all three of the women had received an injection of a liquid material that he had been given by Doctor Sharon Dell. He asked me to analyze the liquid to determine if there was a link between the fluid and the cancers. He suspected that the vial might contain the answer."

"What did you do then?"

"I read the label on the vial and noticed that the top right hand corner of the label was smeared with something. I then made a call to the San Bernardino's Sheriff's Forensic Laboratory."

"Why would you do that?"

Swenz sat up straight upon hearing this latest testimony.

"Well, by nature I am a suspicious person. I have always been intrigued in forensics. As a matter of fact, in addition to my Boards in Pathology and Oncology and my Ph.D. in Genetics, I am also certified by the American Board of Forensic Examiners and the American Board of Forensic Medicine."

"Have you ever done work as a forensic expert?"

"Many times. I have been called as a witness in many cases by various law enforcement agencies to testify about DNA and forensics."

"So, when you were handed the vial by Doctor Herbert and saw the smudged label, you became inquisitive?"

"I wanted to know what the stain was. It might very well have proven helpful. I asked the forensic department to send over a lab tech to lift the stain and test it for me."

"Did they do so?"

"Yes, after I filled out a request form with the department stating my reasons for the request."

"What happened then?"

"Mr. Fred Swartsman came to my office and photographed the vial and then removed some of the label with a scalpel blade. He then tried to absorb part of the stain with a saline solution. He did a quick field test and determined it was blood. The rest of his swab sample was placed into a small glass tube, and he left with the samples. I kept the vial and its contents to analyze."

"Did you eventually arrive at a conclusion as to the material in the vial?" "Yes. It was determined to be an adenovirus that contained an oncogene. That is, a gene that has the ability to cause cancer. The DNA was the same as all three samples from the three women. I located the breast cancer oncogene in the virus, which must have been spliced there previously, and compared it to the DNA oncogene present in the three cancer biopsy samples. They were all identical. All the cancer cells were derived from the same original cancer. This means that someone had to add the oncogene from a breast cancer cell taken from someone else and incorporate it into the virus, which is easy to do today. The virus with the deadly oncogene is injected into the arm and is then trapped at the regional lymph nodes. As the virus is attacked by the body's defenses, the oncogene incorporates itself into the DNA of the person's cells and causes the development of the breast cancer at that site."

The jury looked amazed and so did those watching the trial in the courtroom.

"Did you then discover a method to stop the cancer from growing?"

"Yes, we incorporated a suppressor gene, p53, into an adenovirus and it was injected into the women in the same shoulder. The virus was caught at the same lymph node region as the cancer virus and attacked the breast cancer cells. You see, normal cells all have p53 in their DNA, which codes for a protein that instructs the cancer cell to shut down and die."

Swenz was now livid. "No!" he screamed aloud.

"Another outburst and I will have you removed from the courtroom," exclaimed the judge in annoyance.

"You were saying Doctor ..."

"Well, Doctor Herbert has informed me recently that all the women have tested free of all cancer." He smiled, as did the jury. "May I now direct your attention to the next time you met with Doctor Herbert."

"Yes, about seven weeks ago I met with him, Doctor Sharon Dell, and her father, Doctor Karl Dell. They told me of the plot that had been devised by a Michael Rome to keep Sharon from ever testifying against him and his company."

He referred to the meeting at Spago that Sharon had testified about. Evidently, a microchip had been inserted into a donor liver that was in Karl's abdomen. It was programmed in such a manner that it could begin a process of killing the liver cells when activated. He went on in great detail, explaining how he had foiled the plot by suggesting that the EB Virus be injected into Karl's liver so the Bcl-2 protein produced by this virus would offer permanent protection against liver cell death induction by the microchip.

"Thank you, Doctor. Oh yes, did you ever receive any notice from the sheriff's forensic lab about the smear on the label of the vial you received from Doctor Herbert?"

"Yes. The smear was subjected to DNA analysis and confirmed to be the blood of Doctor Swenz." Swenz became pale.

"As a forensics expert, in your opinion, how does that fit in this picture?"

"Swenz pricked his finger when he tried to withdraw the fluid and accidentally got a drop of blood on the vial. There was a partial fingerprint of his as well, and they also recovered the prints of Sharon Dell and Michael Herbert, in addition to my own. This would indicate that Swenz did indeed bring the vial to Doctor Dell's office and inject her with the cancer virus."

Swenz had his head on the table while his attorney was whispering something in his ear.

"You are dismissed, Doctor." The judge was writing furiously on a legal pad while the courtroom buzzed with excitement. "Doctor Peter Halper," called Acosta. Michael Rome's face drained as he watched Halper being sworn in.

"Doctor, please tell us where you work and what you do." The next few minutes were spent in certifying Peter as an expert witness in genetics. He testified in a forthright manner since he had the DA's assurance that he would be given immunity in return for his extensive statements given to the DA concerning the Research Laboratory and all their involvement with World Health Care HMO and TWMC. He testified that he had created the microchip that could be activated by a computer through the GPS satellite and explained how the process of apoptosis worked. His testimony sealed the outcome for all the conspirators.

"Thank you, Doctor, you may step down."

The defense attempted in vain to restore Swenz's credibility.

The thrust of Mr. Grant's case was to show a conspiracy against Swenz and that there was no attempt to seek help for him to overcome his gambling addiction. There was testimony that strongly showed Swenz was an addict and were it not for the addiction, he would not have fallen prey to those who paid him to do illegal things. However, Grant was hard pressed to show mitigating factors when it came to his act against Sharon.

The jury returned the verdict in two days against Swenz, but a plea bargain was entered by Acosta after the first day of testimony for Michael Rome and David Malkin and their respective companies. The same plea bargains were entered for TWMC and the World Health HMO at that time. The plea bargain called for a five-year sentence for each of the CEOs and a two-million-dollar fine from each of the four conspirators for state violations of the health and welfare code. The jury found Swenz guilty of attempted murder and conspiracy to commit murder. He was sentenced two weeks later to fifteen years at the Chino State Prison.

Michael and Sharon went to dinner, where they talked. Each one probed their mind in an attempt to come to terms with their feelings. They explored their relationship with each other as well as Sharon's involvement with Swenz, the trial, the attacks, and most frightening, the cancer. They both realized the importance of the previous year's events and how they related to the "bigger picture," but the significance of Sharon's role in the program was not yet fully comprehended. They both knew that this was the beginning of a long process and that only time would tell their future.

-45-

THE ENDS JUSTIFY THE MEANS

Andrew Veccia was in his office high atop the Crescent Park Casino when his phone rang.

"Yes, this is Andrew."

"This is Jimmy Drake. I have the information you wanted. Doctor Granatelli is the prison doctor at Chino. I spoke with him last evening. He assures me he has never forgotten his debt to you for what you did years ago for his family."

"That's good! Very good indeed. Tell him we'll be in touch." Andrew dialed another number. "Did you get it?" He smiled and hung up.

A week ago, after he'd added up the amount of money Swenz owed him, Andrew was furious. "He owes me $30,000 and I'm the laughingstock of Vegas. I have my reputation to consider, as well as my pride." He called Tony, who had a friend who worked at the University Hospital. He promised he would take care of it.

Gary could well use a thousand dollars and it would be

easy. He was employed as a housekeeper by the hospital and had all the master keys, which allowed him access to any locked door. Gary was given a small vial, a syringe and needle, and shown how to remove fluid from a vial. After demonstrating his competence in performing the act and receiving information on what to look for, Tony sent him on his way.

That night, when everyone had gone home, he unlocked the door of the Genetic Cancer Lab and then the door of Doctor Kohl's office. Gary rummaged around the private office until he became exasperated. He saw a small refrigerator on the floor under a bench in the corner of the room and opened the door. There, on the top shelf, was a small brown envelope that was labeled Doctor Herbert — DNA. There were about two milliliters left in the vial. He inserted a needle and withdrew one milliliter, then capped the syringe and inserted it into his pocket. He then walked out and locked both doors. When he was alone in the restroom, he removed the needle and syringe and injected its contents into the empty vial he carried in his pocket. When he left the job, he reported his success and rendezvoused with Tony, who handed him an envelope containing ten one-hundred-dollar bills.

▲ ▲ ▲

Swenz had been kept at the County Jail until two days ago, when he was driven to Chino State Prison. He was trying to adjust to the environment.

"You're wanted in Medical," said the guard. He followed the guard from the laundry, where he had been assigned, to the medical ward of the prison. "Sit here," ordered the guard. The guard walked to the nurse's desk and spoke with her for a moment. "Over here," he commanded. Swenz walked to the desk.

"You may go in to see the Doctor now," said the nurse. *I wonder what this is all about*, thought Swenz. He walked through the door to find himself face to face with Doctor Granatelli.

"I am the prison doctor. Feel free to see me if you have any medical problems. He struck an immediate rapport with Swenz that placed Swenz at ease. After spending twenty minutes taking a medical history, which was standard procedure as Granetelli explained, he informed his captive audience that all new prisoners had to receive flu shots to prevent any potential epidemic that was so prevalent in crowded areas. "Roll up your sleeve, please." Swenz rolled his shirt sleeve up and Granetelli gave him the flu shot. "If you need me, I'm here. Good to meet you." Swenz exited and was taken to the laundry again.

It was about two months later when he asked to see Doctor Granetelli.

"What can I do for you, Barry?"

"Will you check this for me? I don't know how I got it, but I feel a large mass here in my armpit."

The End

AUTHOR'S NOTE

I wrote this novel in 1995, when medical genetics was starting to bloom. It was the beginning of gene identification to discover the causes of many inherited diseases. Prior to that time, there was no genetic research development to help doctors choose the appropriate drug to treat a particular disease.

I developed this story about drug manufacturers, genetic research companies, doctors, and hospitals all vying for the almighty buck. I became motivated through my observation of all these entities, watching how they were only interested in money and not in helping the sick. Through the story, I brought to bear genetic realities that have since come to the forefront. The following is an excerpt from the 2016 *Scientific American* article, "20 Years after Dolly the Sheep Led the Way—Where Is Cloning Now?"

> *It was a glorious day in the hills above Edinburgh, Scotland, when old friends and scientific colleagues Ian Wilmut and Alan Trounson set off on a hike two decades ago. High over the city, Wilmut confided that he had a secret to share. As part of a larger study, he and several co-workers had successfully birthed a lamb in the lab—not from egg and sperm but from DNA taken from an adult sheep's mammary gland. They had cloned a mammal. "Crikey, I was stunned," says Trounson, who is*

now—as then—a stem cell biologist at Monash University in Melbourne, Australia. He remembers sitting down hard on a nearby stone. It was a warm day but Trounson felt a chill pass over him as he realized the implications. "It changed everything."

In *Send in the Clones*, I developed my rendition of the cloning procedure at about the same time the true researchers began theirs. This stuns me that actual cloning has occurred today.

I have endeavored to write about all the genetic theories that were available in 1995 with the exception of the literary license in the area of activating a chip in the liver to destroy the liver cells and a few more zones of genetic engineering. In 1995 and now there continues extensive research with EBV and the p53 gene, and BCL2 gene in regulating apoptosis.

All the illnesses, diagnostics and patient evaluations, were drawn from my experiences practicing internal medicine which included teaching nurses and pre-med students. The illnesses and complications occurred in actual patients.

Because liver and kidney transplants were always in such demand, I was driven to create a fictional new source for organ transplants, and thus the cloning in the book. My plot also required a world-wide need for liver transplants, thus creating a pandemic of hepatitis D2. Now, we are in a true pandemic today, which makes this book an exciting, though unfortunately timely, read.

Marvin Ginsburg, MD